ANAESTHESIA
UNCOMMON DIS

This book is dedicated to our wives,
Claire and Gill

Anaesthesia for Uncommon Diseases

B.J. POLLARD
BPharm MB ChB FFARCS
Senior Lecturer in Anaesthesia,
University of Manchester;
Department of Anaesthesia,
Manchester Royal Infirmary,
Manchester

M.J. HARRISON
MB BS FFARCS
Specialist Anaesthetist,
Auckland Hospital,
Auckland,
New Zealand

Blackwell Scientific Publications

OXFORD LONDON EDINBURGH

BOSTON MELBOURNE

© 1989 by
Blackwell Scientific Publications
Editorial Offices:
Osney Mead, Oxford OX2 0EL
   (*Orders*: Tel: 0865 240201)
8 John Street, London WC1N 2ES
23 Ainslie Place, Edinburgh EH3 6AJ
3 Cambridge Center, Suite 208
   Cambridge, Massachusetts 02142, USA
107 Barry Street, Carlton
   Victoria 3053, Australia

First published 1989

Set by Setrite Typesetters,
Hong Kong;
printed and bound in Great Britain
by Billing and Sons Ltd,
Worcester

DISTRIBUTORS

USA
   Year Book Medical Publishers
   200 North LaSalle Street
   Chicago, Illinois 60601
   (*Orders*: Tel: (312) 726−9733)

Canada
   The C.V. Mosby Company
   5240 Finch Avenue East
   Scarborough, Ontario
   (*Orders*: Tel: (416) 298−1588)

Australia
   Blackwell Scientific Publications
   (Australia) Pty Ltd
   107 Barry Street
   (*Orders*: Tel: (03) 347−0300)

British Library
Cataloguing in Publication Data

Pollard, B.J. (Brian James)
   Anaesthesia for uncommon diseases
   1. Medicine. Anaesthesia & analgesia
   I. Title II. Harrison, M.J. (Michael
   John), *1946−*
   617'.96

   ISBN 0−632−02406−2

Contents

PREFACE   vii

MONOGRAPHS A–Z   1

INDEX   265

Preface

When formulating a plan of anaesthesia for a patient with an unusual medical, surgical or anaesthetic problem, it is useful to know whether anaesthesia has been administered previously to a patient with such a problem and with what outcome. Reports of such cases appear in almost every anaesthetic journal, but where do you look to find the article that you want? The aim of this book is to draw together as much of this information as possible and to place that information between two covers. The scope of the book encompasses the anaesthetic literature between 1960 and 1987.

Many disorders are confusing in the plethora of synonyms which exist. These have been kept as straightforward as possible and each monograph headed by a current recognised preferred term [1] followed by a short list of those other names which might be commonly encountered. The original sources of information have been included at the foot of each monograph (where there is a large number of references, a selection only has been included) so that the reader may refer back to them for more details. These references are referred to by numbers in the text if relating to a particular point.

It must be stressed that it is not the intention of this book to describe the only way to tackle a particular problem, but rather to inform the reader whether it has been done before and how it was done. Armed with this information it is then up to the individual anaesthetist to formulate his or her own plan of management. Descriptions of standard techniques, e.g. rapid sequence induction, have not been included. It is important to remember that in view of the complex nature of some medical conditions they are best managed in a specialist unit.

Finally, it should be noted that this is not an exhaustive text. Every effort has been made to trace as many relevant reports as possible but it is inevitable that some have been missed and others described since the book went into production. The authors would therefore appreciate hearing of such omissions so that future editions may thus be rendered more complete.

BJP
MJH

Reference

1 Bergsma D (Ed.) (1979) *Birth Defects Compendium*, 2nd edn. National Foundation March of Dimes, MacMillan, London.

Acanthosis nigricans

Major problem
Friable lesions in mouth and pharynx

Acanthosis nigricans is a rare condition that may either be benign or malignant (about a quarter of cases). There is symmetrical warty hyperplasia of the skin with hyperpigmentation. Lesions may be found around the mouth, on the palate, gums and tongue. Oral lesions are found predominantly in the malignant group and it is this group that will be more likely to present for surgery. In the majority of such patients the primary neoplasm is in the stomach.

The fragile nature of the lesions causes them to bleed and slough when manipulated by oropharyngeal airways, laryngoscopes or tracheal tubes. Great care must therefore be taken with the airway. Consider a regional anaesthetic technique in preference to general anaesthesia whenever possible.

Further reading

McKissic ED. *Anesthesiology*, 1975; **42:** 357−358.

Achondroplasia
Chondrodystrophica fetalis

Major problems
Upper airway difficulty
Spinal cord compression
Thoracolumbar kyphosis
Atlanto-axial instability

Achondroplasia is a dominantly inherited condition characterised by very short limbs, foramen magnum insufficiency and thoracolumbar kyphosis.

During 24 anaesthetics given to 11 patients 'There were no serious complications associated with any of the anaesthetic agents or techniques' [1]. Moderate difficulty with intubation and failure to perform a lumbar puncture were the two problems mentioned. Even though there were no neurological sequelae the authors considered it prudent to avoid spinal anaesthesia. 50% of achondroplastic dwarfs have symptomatic spinal stenosis and the intervertebral discs are prone to bulge laterally and posteriorly; symptomatic herniations, however, are uncommon. Mayhew *et al.* [2] reviewed over 20 patients, many of them undergoing foramen magnum decompression in the sitting position, and described spinal cord infarction and venous air embolism. The intubation difficulty is due to the inability to extend the head on the cervical spine. The atlas lies beneath a concave occiput and the arch of the atlas limits the movement. Equipment for a difficult intubation should be available. Mayhew *et al.* [2] considered the weight of the patient to be the best guide to the size of the tracheal tube.

6−12 kg	4.0−5.0 mm
20−30 kg	6.0−6.5 mm
over 30 kg	7.0 mm

During pregnancy the physiological disturbances that occur are exaggerated: the baby is virtually normal size but the pelvis and abdominal cavity are smaller [3]. There is impaired cardiorespiratory function with a marked reduction in functional residual capacity. There is also greater risk of supine hypotension. Patients should be carefully counselled regarding the problems of both general and local anaesthesia.

References

1 Mather JS. *Anaesthesia,*1966; **21:** 244–248.
2 Mayhew JF, Katz J, Miner M, Leimann BC, Hall ID. *Can. Anaesth. Soc. J.,* 1986; **33:** 216–221.
3 Cohen SE. *Anesthesiology,* 1980; **52:** 264–266.

Further reading

Bancroft GH, Lauria JI. *Anesthesiology,* 1983; **59:** 143–144.
McPherson RW, North RB, Udvarhelyi GB, Rosenbaum AE. *Anesthesiology,* 1984; **61:** 764–767.
Walts LF, Finerman G, Wyatt GM. *Can. Anaesth. Soc. J.,* 1975; **22:** 703–709.

Acromegaly

Major problems
Upper airway difficulty
Multiple endocrine abnormalities including
   glucose intolerance and hypopituitarism

Acromegaly is the result of excessive growth hormone secretion from a pituitary adenoma and this leads to overgrowth of the skeleton and soft tissues. It has an incidence in the population of about 40 : 1 000 000. A large tongue and general tissue thickening of the upper airway are features of acromegaly that may cause the anaesthetist a problem in the form of airway obstruction. The epiglottis, aryepiglottic folds and ventricular folds, vocal cords and arytenoid cartilages may all be thickened. The vocal cords may be fixed. "The anaesthetist who encounters an acromegalic with voice changes should be alerted to the possibility of involvement of larynx with narrowing of the glottic opening" [1]. However, five out of six patients with voice changes, reported by Burn [2], were all successfully intubated and had no postoperative distress. If laryngeal stenosis is present then prophylactic tracheostomy should be considered prior to the removal of the tracheal tube.

Southwick & Katz advocated elective tracheostomy if the patient should exhibit obvious signs of respiratory obstruction, nocturnal dyspnoea, snoring, exertional dyspnoea or stridor [3]. Messick et al., however, anaesthetised 94 acromegalic patients without having to resort to tracheostomy [4], although six patients had to be intubated with the aid of a fibreoptic bronchoscope. The visualisation of the larynx indirectly by mirror may help preoperatively, although failure to visualise the larynx may not indicate a difficult intubation [2].

Hypersomnia with airway obstruction and prolonged breath holding has been described and, following an acute obstruction, acute pulmonary oedema has occurred. The pulmonary oedema was thought to be due to the "relief of the obstruction and consequent increased venous return from the redistribution of intravascular volume from the peripheral to the central circulation" [5].

Other problems associated with the management of patients with acromegaly include hypopituitarism, hyperthyroidism, hyperprolactinaemia, hyperparathyroidism, phaeochromocytoma and carcinoid. Diabetes mellitus, diabetes insipidus (very rare), and heat intolerance due to an increased metabolic rate may also occur. There may in addition be a cardiomyopathy, hypertension, spondylosis, neuropathy (possibly diabetic) and a myopathy.

References

1 Kitahata LM. *Br. J. Anaesth.*, 1971; **43:** 1187–1190.
2 Burn JMB. *Br. J. Anaesth.*, 1972; **44:** 413–414.
3 Southwick JP, Katz J. *Anesthesiology*, 1979; **51:** 72–73.
4 Messick JM, Cucchiara RF, Faust RJ. *Anesthesiology*, 1982; **56:** 157.
5 Goldhill DR, Dalgleish JG, Lake RHN. *Anaesthesia*, 1982; **37:** 1200–1203.

Acute idiopathic polyneuritis

Guillain-Barré syndrome,
Acute infectious polyneuritis

Major problems
Autonomic dysfunction
Possible K$^+$ release with suxamethonium

The Guillain-Barré syndrome is a demyelinating disease process usually presenting as progressive weakness and paraesthesia in the limbs. The weakness may extend proximally to eventually result in quadriplegia with difficulty in swallowing and breathing. Management is symptomatic. The associated autonomic dysfunction can take the form of either excessive or inadequate activity of the sympathetic and/or parasympathetic systems [1]. Postural hypotension occurs in about 40% of patients with the disease. The syndrome can occur, rarely, during a pregnancy and the labile cardiovascular system can make the diagnosis of pre-eclamptic toxaemia difficult. Carbon dioxide tensions during pregnancy should be kept within the physiological range for pregnancy (25–34 mmHg); below this range fetal hypoxia is possible.

Head up tilting is best avoided as the prolonged immobilisation in bed will exaggerate the cardiovascular instability. Any change of position should be carried out with care and the patient continuously monitored. Intermittent positive pressure ventilation may produce peripheral pooling of blood and thus should be implemented with care. If spinal or epidural anaesthesia is contemplated intravascular expansion is necessary even with a low block—blood loss should be replaced promptly. It has been suggested that anaesthetic agents with a sympathomimetic effect should be used and that barbiturates and phenothiazines should be avoided. Continuous comprehensive monitoring is essential. In patients with spinal cord injury, brain injury and motor neurone disease suxamethonium may produce marked hyperkalaemia [2]. Such a response has not so far been observed in the Guillain-Barré syndrome but caution is advisable in any patient with paralytic disease. The vulnerable period is 7—90 days after onset of symptoms.

References

1 Perel A, Reches A, Davidson JT. *Anaesthesia*, 1977; **32:** 257—260.
2 Beach TP, Stone WA, Hamelberg W. *Anesth. Analg.*, 1971; **50:** 431—437.

Further reading

Elstein M, Legg NJ, Murphy M, Park DM, Sutcliffe MML. *Anaesthesia*, 1971; **26:** 216—224.
Smith RB. *Can. Anaesth. Soc. J.*, 1971; **18:** 199—201.

Alveolar proteinosis

Major problems
Lower airway problem
Hypoxia

Alveolar proteinosis results in the obstruction of the lower airways with inspissated proteinaceous material rich in lipids. Pulmonary lavage is the technique of choice to assist the clearance of the casts. General anaesthesia is considered desirable because, although the procedure is not painful, it is quite distressing and with general anaesthesia unilateral lavage is more easily carried out and hypoxia minimised by controlled ventilation.

In an adult an anaesthetic technique is used that involves the administration of a high inspired oxygen concentration, a double lumen endobronchial tube and neuromuscular blockade. Halothane, enflurane and ketamine-diazepam have all been used as the anaesthetic agents. Most patients require a repeat lavage (to the contralateral lung) a week or two later and thus an alternative to halothane is necessary. It is advantageous to know the pre-anaesthetic values of lung volumes. The correct positioning of the double lumen tube can be demonstrated, as described by Blenkarn et al. [1], by the "absence of bubbling and the rising of the water level in a clear submerged tube connected to one channel of the double lumen tube during ventilation of the contralateral lung". With the patient denitrogenated and in a semi-lateral position, with the lung to be treated dependent, the channel serving that lung is opened and expiration permitted. This same channel is then connected to a reservoir of prewarmed 0.9% saline. A volume of saline equivalent to the FRC of that lung is instilled and then "tidal volumes of 500 ml of normal saline were alternately infused and drained by gravity until the effluent had become clear of airway casts, mucopurulent and proteinaceous material" [1]. Up to 40 litres of saline may be used for one procedure. The patients need post-procedure ventilation for several hours, which is carried out using a single lumen

8

tracheal tube. As much saline as possible is removed by suction, physiotherapy and postural drainage. There are many physiological derangements during the lavage—the physiologic shunt doubles with the lavage but is worst during the expiratory phase of the lavage process—it is assumed that during the inspiratory phase the filling of the lung with more fluid compresses the pulmonary vessels and thus reduces the perfusion of the un-ventilated lung. Cardiac output is thought to be reduced due to a reduction in venous return. The monitoring of Pa_{O_2} is essential.

For a similar procedure in children the lack of endobronchial tubes makes the use of extracorporeal circulation mandatory. Using this technique bilateral lung lavage is performed.

Saline has been shown to be effective and facilitates more complete resorption than is possible with higher molecular weight additives that have been used with the saline.

Reference

1 Blenkarn CD, Lanning CF, Kylstra JA. *Can. Anaesth. Soc. J.*, 1975; **22:** 154−163.

Further reading

Busque L. *Can. Anaesth. Soc. J.*, 1977; **24:** 380−389.
Lippmann M, Mok MS, Wasserman K. *Br. J. Anaesth.*, 1977; **49:** 173−177.

Amaurosis congenita

Leber's disease

Major problem
Extremely abnormal sensitivity to sedative agents

Bilateral optic atrophy and nystagmus are found in this inherited sex-linked condition.

The patient described [1] took, or was given, on separate occassions, two tablets of Distalgesic (dextropropoxyphene hydrochloride 65 mg plus paracetamol 650 mg), 5 mg diazepam and 1 g paracetamol and on each occasion required respiratory support. Be prepared to support ventilation during and after anaesthesia. A premedication is best avoided. The use of nitro-prusside should also be avoided because the patient may have an impaired ability to handle its metabolites.

Reference

1 Hunter AR. *Anaesthesia,* 1984; **39:** 781−783.

Amelia

Ectromelia

Major problems
Vascular access limited
Sites for monitoring limited
Airway difficulty

Complete absence of limbs results in a slightly elevated body temperature and may be associated with other anomalies which include upper airway deformities. The estimated incidence of amelia is 1 in 3.5 million.

Blood pressure monitoring is difficult. Direct arterial cannulation may be necessary, suggested sites being the ilio-inguinal artery or the temporal artery (under direct vision). A Doppler probe may be placed over the temporal artery and a cuff inflated around the head to obtain an indirect reading. Venous access may be achieved via the internal or external jugular veins. Preparation should be made for a possible difficult intubation.

Further reading

Heyman HJ, Ivankovitch HD, Shulman M, Miller E, Choudhry YH. *J. Ped. Orthopedics*, 1982; **2:** 299–301.
Tallmeister A, Sheehan MM, Pelton DA. *Can. Anaesth. Soc. J.*, 1986; **33:** 484–487.

American trypanosomiasis

Chagas' disease

Major problems
Bilateral heart failure
Cardiac conduction defects
Achalasia
Autonomic and peripheral neuropathy

This is a disease of North and South America. The infecting organism, *Trypanosoma cruzi*, is carried by blood sucking bugs from mammal to mammal. Millions of the South American population have positive serology, although few have clinical organ damage (Chagas' disease) which occurs decades after the acute phase of infection. There is fragmentation of heart muscle fibres with infiltration by lymphocytes. The Purkinje fibres become inflamed and this leads to conduction disturbances. A similar inflammation occurs in the parasympathetic ganglia.

Digoxin is not always beneficial, and beta-blockade is dangerous. Procainamide and lignocaine are used for extrasystoles and ventricular tachycardia, although both are negative inotropes and should be used with great care in patients with a decompensated cardiomyopathy. The patient may have an implanted pacemaker. Autonomic neuropathy results in a sympathetic predominance and thus as an anti-arrythmic agent bretyllium is recommended because it has no effect on myocardial contractility and also has a sympathetic blocking action. Mega-oesophagus and megacolon occur: the former results in difficulty in swallowing (in its severe form oesophageal contents may spill into the airway and cause repeated chest infections), the latter results in chronic constipation. It is wise to avoid atropine (ventricular irritability), to avoid negative inotropes and to use a neurolept technique. Great care must be taken to avoid respiratory soiling should achalasia be present.

Further reading

De Castro Barreto JC. *Br. J. Anaesth.*, 1979; **51**: 1189.

Amyloidosis

Major problems
Multisystem dysfunction
Skin easily damaged

Amyloidosis, either primary or secondary (classically due to chronic suppurative disease), is the condition that follows the deposition of a glycoprotein in many tissues—the kidney, the liver, the heart—all leading to impairment of function. The skin is not excluded from the process and may be damaged by minimal trauma caused by adhesive tape and ECG electrodes. On removal of the adherent article skin may be stripped, there may be gross ecchymoses and there may be frank bleeding. The bleeding is due to deposition of the amyloid in the small blood vessels. Bullous eruptions may also occur. About 40% of patients with amyloid have skin involvement.

Care should be taken to investigate all major systems: liver, spleen, kidney, heart, lungs, adrenals, pancreas, thyroid, intestine, bladder and skin. It is possible for the larynx to be involved and dominate the symptomatology.

Further reading

Dixon J. *Anaesthesia*, 1987; **42:** 218.
Welch DB. *Anaesthesia*, 1982; **37:** 63−66.

Amyotrophic lateral sclerosis

Motor neurone disease, primary lateral sclerosis, pseudobulbar palsy, progressive muscular atrophy, poliomyelitis

---

Major problems
Hyperkalaemia with suxamethonium
Prolonged paralysis with non-depolarising muscle
relaxants

There are several varieties of motor neurone disease, a demyelinating process, and they have been classified in the following way.
1 Motor cortex and efferent pathways—primary lateral sclerosis.
2 Including brain stem—pseudobulbar palsy.
3 Spinal cord and anterior horn cells—progressive muscular atrophy.

There is progressive muscular atrophy and spasticity due to involvement of the pyramidal tracts. This may be difficult to detect in some patients. Fasciculations, weakness and atrophy are the three hallmarks of the condition. The condition may be associated with an underlying malignancy.

Poliomyelitis is an infectious viral disease which affects the anterior horn cells of the spinal cord and medulla. It is included in this section because of similarities in management.

Hyperkalaemia has been noted to occur in response to suxamethonium, as in other denervation states. The prolonged activity of non-depolarising agents is thought to be due to an abnormality of neuromuscular transmission which seems to exist in those muscle groups affected by the disease—subclinical dysfunction may thus be exposed by the use of non-depolarising agents. Should muscle relaxation be considered necessary it is suggested that small doses of non-depolarising agents be used with neuromuscular function monitoring. Respiratory depressants, including barbiturates, should be given carefully in reduced dosage. Postoperative respiratory support may be necessary. If the bulbar muscles are affected there may be laryngeal incompetence with weakness in swallowing and a weak gag reflex. There is therefore an increased likelihood of tracheal aspiration occurring at any time, including the peri-operative period.

Further reading

Azar I. *Anesthesiology*, 1984; **61:** 173–187.
Beach TP, Stone WA, Hamelberg W. *Anesth. Analg.*, 1971; **50:** 431–437.
Rosenbaum KJ, Neigh JL, Strobel GE. *Anesthesiology*, 1971; **35:** 638–641.

Analgesia — congenital

Major problems
Inadvertent damage to skin/joints
Possible failure of thermoregulation
Possible vasomotor instability

Congenital analgesia is a hereditary sensory and autonomic neuropathy. It is a rare condition which may be associated with anhydrosis. Fingers, feet and joints suffer the greatest damage resulting from the lack of sensation. The patient may be mentally retarded. Abnormal differentiation of the neural crest or a development defect within the nervous system have been suggested as possible causes. Catecholamine levels are low.

The need for analgesia is absent, although it is possible that there may be islands of tissue with normal sensitivity. Amputations may be carried out with sedation alone—these are the most common procedures as indolent ulcers fail to heal and joints become destroyed. General anaesthesia may be required if the patient is uncooperative. Care over the maintenance of blood volume and the minimal use of vaso-active agents will diminish the effects of the autonomic neuropathy. Atropine is best avoided if anhydrosis exists and a cooling blanket should be available. The operating table should be well padded to prevent inadvertent skin damage and joints should be carefully positioned.

Further reading

Layman PR. *Anaesthesia*, 1986; **41**: 395–397.
Mitaka C, Tsunoda Y, Hikawa Y, Sakahira K, Matsumoto I. *Anesthesiology*, 1985; **63**: 328–329.

Ankylosing spondylitis

Marie Strumpell arthritis

Major problems
Limited head/neck movement
Limited mouth opening
Restrictive pulmonary defect

This progressive inflammatory arthritis of the spine affects males more than females with a peak incidence in the third and fourth decades. Backache and stiffness, worse in the mornings, progresses to marked stiffness and rigidity of the whole of the spine. In advanced cases the whole vertebral column may be fused into one solid structure. Decreased movement of the costovertebral joints results in a reduction in chest movement and consequently a restrictive pulmonary function disorder.

The problems associated with general anaesthesia are those of the maintenance of the airway. The head may be fixed in a flexed position with limited mouth opening. Flexion may be so severe that access to the neck for elective (or emergency) tracheostomy is minimal or even impossible. The arytenoid cartilages may be involved in the inflammatory process.

Awake intubation should be seriously considered. Blind nasal intubation may be tried but may cause trauma with subsequent difficulty in maintaining the airway. A fibreoptic bronchoscope, passed through the tracheal tube or through a nostril and thus used to aid positioning of the tube, may solve the problem. Spinal and epidural anaesthesia are usually not possible because of the ossification of the interspinous ligaments. Pulmonary function tests should be performed as part of the routine preoperative assessment.

Further reading

De Board JW, Ghia JN, Guilford WB. *Anesthesiology*, 1981; **54:** 164–166.

Anomalous lung

Major problem
Hypoxia, infection

The lungs and oesophagus develop from a common embryonic structure and abnormal communications may occasionally form. In all cases described where a main bronchus has originated from the oesophagus it has always been on the right side. The definitive treatment is pneumonectomy with a gastrostomy. Other congenital abnormalities are usually present. Recurrent chest infection, consolidation, pyothorax and pyrexia result.

Pus may be regurgitated and swallowed—assume a full stomach. The following points should be observed:

1 Empty the stomach with suction pre-induction.

2 There may be a blind pouch where the right main bronchus should be and thus the tracheal tube should not be advanced too far.

3 The procedure is best performed in the supine position as in the lateral position, with the pyothorax uppermost, there is a greater risk of the regurgitation of pus and mediastinal shift.

Further reading

Mukai S, Kikuchi H, Akiyama H, Morio M. *Br. J. Anaesth.*, 1977; **49**: 379–382.

Aortic arch abnormalities

Major problems
Chest infection
Hypoxia

Some anomalies of the aortic arch may lead to compression of the trachea or oesophagus—others may be entirely asymptomatic. The symptoms with which the patient presents will depend on the lesion but stridor, dyspnoea, recurrent respiratory infection and feeding difficulties or vomiting may be indicators for radiological investigation. Vascular rings that enclose the trachea and oesophagus tighten with growth. Tracheomalacia and bronchomalacia occur.

Postoperative secretion control may be a problem. Intubation and ventilation may be necssary to maintain good gaseous exchange and to facilitate tracheobronchial toilet.

Further reading

Del Pizzo A. *Br. J. Anaesth.*, 1969; **41**: 898–903.

Apnoea — obstructive sleep

Sleep apnoea syndrome: includes the Pickwickian syndrome, central alveolar hypoventilation, primary alveolar hypoventilation and Ondine's curse

---

Major problems
Airway obstruction—hypoxia
Systemic/pulmonary hypertension
Dysrhythmias

A ten-second apnoea occurring at least thirty times during sleep hours is sufficient for the diagnosis of this condition. Some patients may stop breathing hundreds of times and for periods of up to 90 seconds. The vast majority of the patients have an obstructed upper airway, the remainder have a central respiratory drive deficiency or have a mixed condition. Patients with this syndrome are more likely to suffer postoperative respiratory arrests—the group of patients in whom the risk of the condition existing is greater include diabetics with autonomic neuropathy, patients with micrognathia, myotonic dystrophy and kyphoscoliosis. There are many conditions that pre-dispose to sleep apnoea. A number of patients with alveolar hypoventilation are grossly obese (see p. 178).

Avoid pre-operative and postoperative sedation. Lamarche *et al.* [1] used epidural morphine for postoperative analgesia and their patient developed severe respiratory depression 8 hours later. Airway control may be difficult during induction (pre-oxygenate) and intubation of the trachea may not be straightforward. Ventilation should be controlled, particularly in those patients with a central respiratory drive dysfunction. This also minimises the dose of depressant agents that are required. Postoperatively patients should be monitored with a pulse oximeter to detect desaturation of the blood due to an apnoeic episode. Postoperative analgesia is best provided using a local anaesthetic technique. Excessive oxygen therapy is controversial: the apnoeic episodes may be prolonged and result in a greater level of hypercarbia and acidosis; however, hypoxaemia may be less. Progesterone therapy has been reported to lower the Pa_{CO_2} in these patients [2].

Elective tracheostomy should be considered in those patients who are thought to be at great risk and in whom an emergency tracheostomy may be difficult, for example the extremely obese. The pharynx and larynx may be assessed by a transnasal fibreoptic instrument. It is advisable to secure the airway with a tracheal tube before performing tracheostomy. Tracheostomy, or relief of the airway by any means, does not ensure adequate ventilation—decreased airway resistance is associated with decreased respiratory drive—and as such may exacerbate an already deficient central dysfunction.

Secondary changes which may occur in response to the repeated airway obstruction are systemic and pulmonary hypertension. These may lead to right heart failure and cardiac dysrhythmias. If the cause of the apnoea is a functional disorder of the pharyngeal musculature then uvulopalatopharyngoplasty may help the patient.

References

1 Lamarche Y, Martin R, Reiher J, Blaise G. *Can. Anaesth. Soc. J.*, 1986; **33:** 231−233.
2 McKenzie R, Wadhwa RK. *Anesth. Analg.*, 1977; **56:** 133−135.

Further reading

Chung F, Crago RR. *Can. Anaesth. Soc. J.*, 1982; **29:** 439−445.
Haavik PE. *Can. Anaesth. Soc. J.*, 1983; **30:** 317−318.
Hargrave SA, Legge JS, Palmer KNV. *Br. J. Anaesth.*, 1973; **45:** 111−112.
Newman GC, Baldwin CC, Petrini AJ, Wise L, Wollman SB. *Anesth. Analg.*, 1986; **65:** 985−987.
Rafferty TD, Ruskis A, Sasaki C, Gee JB. *Br. J. Anaesth.*, 1980; **52:** 619−622.
Spector M, Bourke DL. *Anesthesiology*, 1977; **46:** 296−297.
Tseuda K, Shibutani K, Lefkowitz M. *Anesth. Analg.*, 1975; **54:** 523−526.

Apudomas

Multiple endocrine adenomatosis, insulinoma,
Zollinger-Ellison syndrome, vipomas,
Wermer's syndrome, Werner-Morrison syndrome,
WDHA syndrome, Sipple's syndrome

Major problems
Depend upon hormones involved
Rapid changes in blood pressure likely

APUD cells are so named because they possess the capability for
Amine Precursor Uptake and Decarboxylation. They are present
throughout the body in association with many glandular structures. A tumour of a particular APUD cell line is an apudoma
and its particular presentation depends upon the endocrine
hormones produced. Gastrin is produced in excess from a gas-
trinoma (Zollinger-Ellison syndrome), glucagon from a glucagonoma (see page 92), vaso-active intestinal polypeptide (VIP)
from a vipoma (Werner-Morrison syndrome, WDHA syndrome)
[1] and insulin from an insulinoma (see page 115). There are
two syndromes designated multiple endocrine adenomatosis
(MEA) I and II, where hyperparathyroidism (see page 111) resulting from a parathyroid adenoma is associated with either a
pituitary adenoma (MEA I, Wermer's syndrome) or a medullary
carcinoma of the thyroid gland and a phaeochromocytoma (see
page 199) (MEA II, Sipple's syndrome).

Anaesthetic management depends principally on the nature of
the endocrine hormone in excess. Full pre-operative assessment
of the patient with respect to this point is necessary. Many of the
tumours secrete a vasoactive substance and it is therefore advisable to have agents for rapid control of hypotension or hypertension readily to hand. The surgeon should attempt to handle the
tumour as little as possible until the venous supply has been
ligated. Rapid changes in blood pressure may follow the removal
of the tumour and for this reason the insertion of an arterial line
is recommended. There are no anaesthetic drugs or techniques
which are contraindicated with the possible exception of suxa-

methonium. If the tumour is intra-abdominal the transient increase in intra-abdominal pressure which may follow the administration of suxamethonium might liberate hormone into the
circulation.

Reference

1 Taylor AR, Chulajaha D, Jones DH, Whitwam JG. *Anaesthesia*, 1977; **32:** 1012–1016.

Arachnodactyly

Marfan's syndrome

Major problem
Cardiac dysrhythmia

Arachnodactyly is a relatively rare disorder (4−6:100 000) which has an autosomal dominant pattern of inheritance with incomplete expressivity. The primary defect is in elastic tissue—connective tissue strength is decreased and elasticity increased.

Those features of importance to the anaesthetist include mitral and aortic regurgitation, kyphoscoliosis, pectus carinatum, pectus excavatum, high arched palate, laxity of joints and reduced muscle tone. Aortic dilatation may cause tracheal compression. The most common surgery undertaken is for scoliosis and for the cardiovascular lesions. Mortality is high during or following surgery (5−15%). Dysrhythmias are the commonest cause of death, followed by pulmonary complications. Difficulty in tracheal intubation is not a normal feature of the syndrome.

Further reading

Mesrobian RB, Epps JL. *Anesth. Analg.*, 1986; **65**: 411−413.
Verghese C. *Anaesthesia*, 1984; **39**: 917−922.
Woolley MM, Morgan S, Hays DH. *J. Ped. Surg.*, 1967; **2**: 325−331.

Arthrogryposis multiplex congenita

Major problem
Possible airway difficulty

Arthrogryposis multiplex congenita is possibly the result of both muscular and neuromuscular abnormalities—these result in joint fixation and muscle contractures which are present at birth.

In three children out of a series of 67 intubation was found to be difficult. Hypoplasia of the mandible and cleft palate were two noted abnormalities. Of these 67 patients 45 had received multiple halothane anaesthesia without adverse reaction. The risk of malignant hyperpyrexia has been suggested—it would appear not to be proven.

Further reading

Baines DR, Douglas ID, Overton JH. *Anaesth. Intensive Care,* 1986; **14:** 370–372.

Friedlander HL, Westin GW, Wood WL. *J. Bone Joint Surg.,* 1968; **50A:** 89–112.

Itohda Y. *Masui,* 1976; **25:** 697–703.

Asymmetrical septal hypertrophy

Idiopathic hypertrophic subaortic stenosis (IHSS)

Major problem
Possible failure of cardiac output

This is a hypertrophic cardiomyopathy with asymmetrical septal hypertrophy as the common finding. It is transmitted as an autosomal dominant trait. To avoid obstruction, myocardial contractility should be kept at normal or subnormal levels, the preload should not be allowed to fall (hypovolaemia or raised intrathoracic pressure) and neither should the afterload. Myocardial ischaemia is likely. Propranolol, verapamil and nifedipine are all beneficial. Digitalis, isoprenaline, nitroglycerine and amyl nitrate should all be avoided.

Halothane is acceptable. Using a narcotic/muscle relaxant/nitrous oxide anaesthetic technique it was shown that the addition of 0.25% halothane had a beneficial effect in shortening the systolic time interval QF [1] (this is the time in msecs from the Q wave of the ECG to the upstroke of the peripheral pulse). There was no overt change in blood pressure or heart rate. Isoflurane and enflurane are not so good—the systemic vascular resistance is reduced. Spinal and epidural block are not advised for similar reasons. Methoxamine and phenylephrine are the vasopressors of choice, having no direct cardiac effects. Ergometrine is preferable to oxytocin in the third stage of labour.

In pregnancy, the blood volume is increased but the systemic vascular resistance is decreased. Aorto-caval compression can cause a reduction in preload and the exertion during labour releases catecholamines and could, together with the inevitable Valsalva manoeuvres, cause problems. Beta blockade is not advocated throughout pregnancy because of adverse effects on the fetus but it is useful during labour.

Reference

1 Reitan JA, Wright RG. *Can. Anaesth. Soc. J.*, 1982; **29**: 154–157.

Athlete's heart

Major problem
Abnormal vagal sensitivity

Athletes may have an extraordinarily slow heart rate. On induction of anaesthesia the rate may decrease further. Other ECG abnormalities may be noticed, 1st degree and 2nd degree heart block, AV-junctional rhythms, tall peaked T waves and ST elevation. The Wenkebach phenomenon (Mobitz type 1) is a benign dysrhythmia in athletes. Both right and left ventricular hypertrophy may occur but these do not indicate organic disease. Right ventricular hypertrophy may result in ECG changes of right bundle branch block. The abnormal vagal sensitivity seems to be restricted to the heart and is probably due to local changes in the myocardium. These changes can take place in as little as six weeks from the onset of training.

These patients should be monitored for even the most minor procedure. Atropine must be available.

Further reading

Abdulatif M, Fahkry M, Naguib M, Gyamfi YA, Saeed I. *Can. J. Anaesth.*, 1987; **34:** 284–287.
Bullock RE, Hall RJC. *Anaesthesia*, 1985; **40:** 647–650.

Auto erythrocyte sensitisation syndrome

Painful bruising syndrome

Major problem
Severe bruising

This is a rare syndrome in which a bruise may occur spontaneously or secondary to minimal trauma. The bruise may be extensive and a haematoma may form. Coagulation studies are normal. A typical reaction can be reproduced by the intradermal injection of autologous red cells. Psychological problems are common in these patients and it has been suggested that there is psychogenic activation of substances causing vascular changes.

Inhalational induction of anaesthesia should be considered. Excessive postoperative surgical bleeding has not been reported; the patient reported had no bruising at the shoulder which was manipulated but had extensive bruising following the atraumatic venepuncture.

Further reading

Hales P. *Anaesth. Intensive Care*, 1981; **9:** 390–391.

Autonomic hyperreflexia

Mass reflex

Major problem
Vascular instability

Autonomic hyperreflexia occurs in quadriplegic and paraplegic patients if the lesion is above T7. The major disturbance is that of extraordinarily high blood pressure. Vagal influences on the heart are intact and so a bradycardia results. Other features include piloerection, sweating and facial flushing. The severe hypertension can cause headache, unconsciousness and convulsions. The response is thought to be due to spinal reflexes which are uninhibited from higher centres. These reflexes are initiated by stimulation below the level of the cord transection and include distension and contraction of the gut, bladder and uterus. The isolated adrenal medulla releases catecholamines and causes a further sympathetic response because of the supersensitive vascular system.

Spinal reflexes can be blocked by epidural anaesthesia; the analgesic component is not actually required. The block due to a subarachnoid injection of local anaesthetic is unpredictable and some hypotension may result—spinals are thus perhaps best avoided. Autonomic hyperreflexia has also been prevented by deep halothane anaesthesia. Bladder distension should be prevented by catheterisation because this acts as a potent trigger for autonomic hyperreflexia. Ganglion blocking agents should be available for the management of hypertension. Maintain an adequate blood volume.

Further reading

Stirt JA, Marco A, Conklin KA. *Anesthesiology*, 1979; **51:** 560−562.

Bartter's syndrome

Major problems
Hypokalaemia
Metabolic alkalosis

This is a syndrome in which the primary defect is uncertain. It may be in the renal tubules, a possible sequence of events being sodium loss stimulating renin secretion, which releases aldosterone which causes hypokalaemia and hyperprostaglandinism. It is probably inherited by an autosomal recessive gene. Drug management includes propranolol to reduce renin release, spironolactone (aldosterone antagonist), and inhibition of prostaglandin synthesis by a non-steroidal anti-inflammatory agent. Angiotensin converting enzyme inhibitors may also be used.

Intra-operatively the patient's electrolyte and acid-base status should be measured regularly. There may be a diuresis both intra-operatively and postoperatively, therefore fluid replacement requirements should be frequently assessed. Hyperventilation should be avoided because of these patients' tendency to metabolic alkalosis. The patients are usually normotensive but their cardiovascular responses to hypovolaemia may be impaired—they are resistant to catecholamines and are likely to be beta-blocked. They appear to excrete drugs adequately through the kidneys. Potassium supplementation is usually required.

Further reading

Abston PA, Priano LL. *Anesth. Analg.*, 1981; **60:** 764–766.

Behçet's syndrome

This disorder belongs amongst the muco-cutaneous ocular syndromes and the manifestations include buccal ulceration, thrombophlebitis and cardiovascular lesions. Ocular and genital lesions also occur but are of less significance to the anaesthetist. It is a chronic disease which ultimately results in blindness—if neurological symptoms develop then dementia and death occur earlier.

Pharyngeal scarring is not common but does occur and may make tracheal intubation extremely difficult. Enquiries should be made for a history of dysphagia and the upper airway examined closely. Avoid trauma to the skin and mucous membranes. Steroid therapy may need reinforcing.

Further reading

Turner ME. *Br. J. Anaesth.*, 1972; **44:** 100–102.

Bilirubin metabolism— abnormalities

Crigler-Najjar types 1 and 2, Dubin Johnson,
Rotor and hepatic storage disease
and Gilbert's syndrome

Major problems
Jaundice/kernicterus
Reduced drug detoxification

Disorders of bilirubin metabolism range from the benign (Gilbert's, Dubin-Johnson, Rotor and hepatic storage disease) through a disease of medium severity (Crigler-Najjar type 2) to the most severe (Crigler Najjar type 1).

Crigler-Najjar type 1

Kernicterus occurs in infancy and death is usual in the first year of life. It is an autosomal recessive condition which has its defect in the conjugation of bilirubin—there is an absence of UDP-glucuronyl transferase. There is gross unconjugated hyperbilirubinaemia and the only treatments are phototherapy and liver transplantation. Hypoxia, acidosis, hyperthermia or hypoglycaemia all increase the risk of kernicterus and thus should be avoided.

Crigler-Najjar type 2

These patients have some UDP-glucuronyl transferase activity but well below normal levels. Neurological damage is rare but may be initiated by hypoxia or infection.

Dubin-Johnson, Rotor and hepatic storage disease

These are relatively benign conditions in which there is conjugated hyperbilirubinaemia which is due to a failure of bilirubin glucuronide transport to the canaliculi. No treatment is required.

Gilbert's syndrome

Unconjugated hyperbilirubinaemia in an otherwise normal patient should suggest Gilbert's syndrome—it probably has an autosomal dominant pattern of inheritance and its incidence may be as high as 6% although its unmasking following surgery is much less common. The defect appears to be a failure in uptake by the liver cells and some failure of conjugation. UDP-glucuronyl transferase activity is reduced.

Factors that cause an increase in unconjugated bilirubin levels are stress, infection and starvation. There may be decreased detoxification of morphine; morphine is normally conjugated to morphine 3-monoglucuronide, because of the sharing of the same metabolic pathway. It is a diagnosis that should be considered if jaundice occurs in the postoperative period.

Further reading

Mowat AP. *Hospital Update*, 1985; **11:** 921–930.
Nishimura TG, Jackson SH, Cohen SJ. *Can. Anaesth. Soc. J.*, 1973; **20:** 709–712.
Taylor S. *Anaesthesia*, 1984; **39:** 1222–1224.

Bone marrow failure

Pancytopenia, myelofibrosis, leucopenia,
anaemia, thrombocytopenia

Major problems
Reduced oxygen carriage
Lowered resistance to infection
Coagulopathy

Bone marrow failure may be the result of many different processes, e.g. marrow infiltration from myelofibrosis, leukaemia, metastatic malignancy, toxicity from drugs, chemicals or radiation. The clinical picture seen depends upon the elements involved, not all of which may be similarly affected. In the case of all of these patients it is wise to seek the advice of a haematologist before commencing anaesthesia or surgery.

Reduction in the red cell mass reduces the oxygen carriage and also reduces the buffering capacity of the blood. A lower limit of 10 g dl^{-1} of haemoglobin in blood is usually accepted for anaesthesia, although it may be necessary to anaesthetise patients with levels lower than 10 g dl^{-1} under certain circumstances (leukaemic patients undergoing therapy, renal failure). Consideration should be given to transfusing the patient before surgery. An increased inspired oxygen concentration (say 50%) during anaesthesia is only of limited value. Potential hypoxaemic episodes in the peri-operative period should be prevented by pre-oxygenation and the administration of oxygen in the immediate postoperative period.

Reduction in the white cell numbers or function renders the patient at increased risk of infection. All procedures, including intubation, should be undertaken with strict attention to asepsis. The use of a sterile disposable anaesthetic circuit may be considered.

Reduction in the platelet numbers or function will increase the patient's bleeding potential. These patients bruise easily and may bleed into joints or body spaces and so great care must be taken when handling them. Intramuscular injections should be avoided and all venepunctures or other instrumentation under-taken with extreme care. An inhalational induction of anaesthesia is useful in these patients. Peri-operative transfusion of platelets may be needed.

Further reading

Bruce DL, Koepke JA. *Anesth. Analg.*, 1972; **51:** 597–605.

Branched chain ketonuria

Maple-syrup urine disease

Major problems
Hypoglycaemia
Acidosis

The frequency of this disease is about 1:250 000. There is a defect in the metabolism of branched chain amino-acids to branched chain fatty acids so that the amino-acids accumulate in the circulation. The branched chain amino-acids valine, leucine and isoleucine are found in many foodstuffs, which have to be restricted, and in body tissues. Following surgery body tissues are broken down and thus there is an acute, potentially lethal, accumulation of these chemicals. Similar events may follow an infection. The patients are slightly mentally retarded and may have some neurological symptoms.

The accumulation of leucine can cause a lowering of the blood glucose and a glucose infusion is therefore mandatory together with regular blood glucose estimations. Postoperative nutrition should be supported by parenteral means in an attempt to reduce body catabolism. Blood in the gastro-intestinal tract may also cause excessive amino-acid absorption. This possibility should be remembered and appropriate measures taken. Not only are the branched chain amino-acids involved in this defect but so are the alpha-keto acids. These are produced from the branched chain amino-acids by oxidative transamination and their presence results in acidosis. Regular pH measurements are important and bicarbonate should be used to correct any derangement. Infection can be lethal.

Further reading

Delaney A, Gal TJ. *Anesthesiology*, 1976; **44**: 83−86.

Buerger's disease

Major problem
Absence of peripheral pulses

Buerger's disease is an occlusive vascular disease which affects the small and medium sized vessels of the extremities. The disease is found in young males and is associated with the smoking of tobacco.

Normally, blood pressure recordings would be taken using a noninvasive method and the patient kept warm to avoid vasospasm due to cold, thus exacerbating the poor peripheral perfusion. If direct arterial pressure monitoring is required then the technique described by Yacoub *et al.* [1] should be considered. The disease process does not usually affect proximal arteries thus axillary artery cannulation was performed after the institution of a continuous brachial plexus block, using the axillary approach. This produced a sympathetic block that increased blood flow to the arm and thus offered some protection against ischaemic damage. It is probably wise to avoid more than minimal hypotension in these patients because of their poor peripheral perfusion.

Reference

1 Yacoub OF, Bacaling JH, Kelly M. *Br. J. Anaesth.*, 1987; **59**: 1056−1058.

Bullous lung disease

Major problems
Maintaining ventilation
Avoiding pneumothorax

Giant bullae usually occur in patients with longstanding chronic obstructive airway disease, thus these patients present with the problems peculiar to the lesion superimposed on those of chronic respiratory dysfunction. Progressive dyspnoea, inability to maintain a normal walking pace on level ground and bullae occupying at least 25% of one hemithorax are the criteria for selecting patients for surgery. The bullae may be of three types: widely open to the bronchi, a narrow opening to the bronchi or those with a ball-valve mechanism.

There are several 'golden' rules:
1 Avoid intermittent positive pressure ventilation if possible—risk of tension pneumothorax.
2 Avoid nitrous oxide—it may diffuse into the bulla and cause it to enlarge.
3 Use a double lumen endobronchial tube so that should spontaneous ventilation be inadequate the bullous lung can be isolated from the 'good' lung and only the good lung ventilated.
Hasenbos and Gielen [1] used a high extradural block using a catheter technique (T3−4) and 0.25% bupivicaine to maintain motor function. They also used gamma-hydroxybutyric acid and droperidol to induce sleep and intubated the patient with a double lumen tube, using a local anaesthetic spray to the cords, and they allowed the patient to breathe 100% oxygen during the thoracotomy.

The local anaesthetic block allowed bronchial suction without distress or cardiovascular response and was effective in preventing bronchospasm. Postoperative analgesia was supplied by the same route using a narcotic. Normandale and Feneck [2] used a high frequency jet ventilator for their patient with a bulla, who was undergoing coronary artery bypass grafting. They used settings of: respiratory rate 250 min^{-1}, volume of driving gas

18 l min^{-1}, inspiratory time 30% of total respiratory cycle and an inspired oxygen of 80%. Anaesthesia was maintained without nitrous oxide and the patient was paralysed. The peak airway pressure is less when a jet ventilator is used.

References

1 Hasenbos MAWM, Gielen MJM. *Anaesthesia*, 1985; **40:** 977−980.
2 Normandale JP, Feneck RO. *Anaesthesia*, 1985; **40:** 1182−1185.

Further reading

Isenhower N, Cucchiara RF. *Anesth. Analg.*, 1976; **55:** 750−752.

Carcinoid syndrome

Major problems
Potential for gross cardiovascular instability
Possible glucose intolerance

Carcinoid tumours have their origins in enterochromaffin cells and release vasoactive substances into the circulation. The cardiovascular response to these agents can be catastrophic. Since 1973 there have been many papers describing the polypharmacy used in an attempt to modifty the action of the released hormones. A pharmaceutical newcomer, somatostatin, seems to make this approach obsolete. Somatostatin prevents the release of the agents from the tumour.

By using the longer-acting analogues of somatostatin and by avoiding agents that trigger the release of the vasoactive substances (drugs that have a tendency to release histamine and adrenergic agents—including endogenous catecholamines released by stress or anxiety) then the hazards associated with anaesthesia in these patients are minimal. Stress is minimised by maintaining normothermia, normovolaemia, normotension and normocapnoea. Somatostatin and its analogues have been termed the 'endocrine cyanide'—insulin release is inhibited and therefore glucose intolerance occurs. Somatostatin has not been proven effective in hypertensive crises and for this situation ketanserin, which is a serotonin antagonist and alpha-adrenergic blocker, is recommended.

Further reading

Roy RC, Carter RF, Wright PD. *Anaesthesia*, 1987; **42**: 627–632.

Cherubism

Hereditary fibrous dysplasia of the jaws
Other synonyms: familial multilocular cystic disease,
bilateral giant cell tumours, familial fibrous swellings,
familial intraosseous fibrous swellings,
familial fibrous dysplasia, familial osseous dysplasia

Major problem
Possible intubation difficulty

The main feature of this rare autosomal dominant, familial disease is mandibular enlargement giving the patient the typical cherubic appearance. This is a disease of childhood and the bony changes are those of cyst formation and hypertrophy. The maxilla may also be involved. Regression of the process occurs in puberty.

Intubation is difficult because of the hypertrophied rami of the mandibles limiting the space available in the mouth for displacement of the tongue. A blind nasal intubation was the successful technique in the case described [1]. The larynx could not be visualised.

Reference

1 Maydew RP, Berry FA. *Anesthesiology*, 1985; **62**: 810−812.

Cholinesterase deficiency (absence)

Major problem
Prolonged paralysis

Pseudocholinesterase (plasma cholinesterase) is produced by the liver and the amounts present can be reduced by a number of conditions including liver disease, malnutrition and pregnancy. Organophosphorus poisoning can also lead to a deficit. A reduced enzyme activity can be found in otherwise healthy individuals and may be due to an atypical enzyme or, more rarely, complete absence of the enzyme. Suxamethonium is hydrolysed by the enzyme and thus an absence of the enzyme results in prolonged paralysis.

With complete absence of the enzyme, elimination of the drug from the neuromuscular endplates is achieved by redistribution and renal excretion. Alkaline hydrolysis of suxamethonium in vivo is very slow. The shortest duration of paralysis reported with complete absence of the enzyme is 2½ hours; the longest 9 hours after using 40 mg suxamethonium. Management is simple —maintain ventilation and sedation until neuromuscular blockade has recovered. The patient's enzyme status and that of the patient's relatives should subsequently be investigated, and the patient advised accordingly.

Further reading

Doenicke A, Gurthner J, Kreutzberg G, Remes I, Speiss W, Steinbereithner K. *Acta Anaesthesiol. Scand.*, 1963; **7**: 59−68.
Dykes MHM, Cheng SC, Valle RF. *Can. Anaesth. Soc. J.*, 1986; **33**: 657−661.
Hart SM, Mitchell JV. *Br. J. Anaesth.*, 1962; **34**: 207−209.

Chondrodystrophia calcificans congenita

Dysplasia epiphysalis punctata, Conradi's syndrome

Major problem
Possible airway problems

This is a rare condition which has an autosomal recessive inheritance. There are consistent signs and there are variable signs of the syndrome—saddle nose deformity, hypertelorism, frontal bossing, high arched palate, short neck and short stature are constant.

The most important functional disorders that are found in some patients are renal and cardiac anomalies and psychomotor retardation. Other signs are flexion contractures, dislocated hips and rhizomelia or micromelia.

Further reading

Nelson MA. *Ann. R. Coll. Surg. Engl.*, 1970; **47:** 185−210.
Tasker WG, Mastri AG, Gold AP. *Am. J. Dis. Child.*, 1970; **119:** 122−127.

Chronic lymphoedema of face

Major problem
Potential airway difficulty

Chronic lymphoedema may be the result of tumour blocking lymphatics, as the result of fibrosis following infection or it may be due to an insufficient number of lymphatics available. The patient described [1] had had a facial infection many years previously and presented with a chronically swollen face—he snored loudly at night.

On induction of anaesthesia the airway was difficult to maintain and on direct laryngoscopy the epiglottis and arytenoid cartilages were found to be swollen. Beware the patient with a swollen face who snores.

Reference

1 Mucklow RG. *Anaesthesia*, 1964; **19:** 570–572.

Coarctation of the aorta (neonatal)

Major problems
Left and right heart failure
Systemic poor perfusion
Multisystem dysfunction

This abnormality accounts for about 7% of congenital cardiovascular lesions. Systemic perfusion may be maintained if the ductus arteriosus remains patent; this delays the diagnosis. The abnormality is associated with hypoplasia of the left heart, ventricular septal defects and miscellaneous other abnormalities of the heart.

A reduction in mortality and morbidity has been achieved by intensive pre-operative preparation—controlled ventilation of the lungs with positive end expiratory pressure, dopamine infusion and prostaglandin E_1 infusion if the ductus needs opening. Prostaglandin E_1 may cause extensive vasodilatation which will necessitate blood volume expansion and it also increases the susceptibility to infection. It reduces the afterload and when used in combination with dopamine, increasing myocardial contractility, it produces a much more efficient pumping action. If systemic hypoperfusion is severe metabolic acidosis and oliguria will result, the former should be treated with sodium bicarbonate and the latter may be improved by the administration of colloid, thus improving blood volume and mean arterial pressure. Arterial and central venous pressures should be monitored directly. Mortality is about 30%.

Further reading

Jones RDM, Duncan AE, Mee RBB. *Anaesth. Intensive Care*, 1985; **13**: 311– 318.

Cockayne's syndrome

Major problems
Potential airway difficulty
Multisystem involvement

This is an autosomal recessive disorder. The main features are those of severely retarded physical development—the nine-year-old described [1] had the appearance and intellect of a three-year-old. Intracranial calcification had resulted in an ataxia and an intention tremor. Elbow and hip contractures had occurred and there was a bony maldevelopment with osteoporosis. Deafness, optic atrophy (which may lead to blindness) and a mixed neuropathy all may be present. Photosensitivity is common. The patient described also had an allergic diathesis.

The problem that this patient presented was of a small-sized maxilla/mandible with normal-sized permanent teeth causing a restriction in the space available for laryngoscopy. Intubation proved difficult but was eventually accomplished. There was a narrowing at the cricoid level and a size 3.5 mm tracheal tube had to be passed before intubation was acceptable.

Reference

1 Cook S. *Anaesthesia*, 1982; **37**: 1104–1107.

Congenital complete heart block

Major problems
Potential inability to respond to cardiovascular
  changes
Associated cardiac lesions

This is a rare conduction defect and may be found in otherwise
perfectly healthy individuals. Other congenital abnormalities
may be present—transposition of the great vessels, single ventricle or a ventricular septal defect. The greatest danger is that of
the patient not responding appropriately to sudden vasodilatation or hypovolaemia. Negative inotropic and chronotropic
agents should be avoided and the facility to pace the heart
should be available.

Ketamine, gallamine and trichloroethylene were all used in
the anaesthetic for the patient described [1]. Atropine was used
as the premedicant together with pethidine, which has an atropine-
like action. Neostigmine should be given with care without
hypoxia or hypercarbia being present. Isoprenaline was held in
readiness. It was suggested that as elective insertion of a pacemaker has its own hazards, these risks should be weighed against
the benefits in an otherwise fit, healthy patient. The indications
suggested for elective insertion of the pacemaker were: 'Stokes-
Adams attacks, no chronotropic response to atropine, QRS interval of more than 0.1 second, exercise intolerance, history of
congestive failure or co-existent cardiac lesion' [2].

References

1 Duffy BL. *Anaesthesia*, 1981; **36:** 956−957.
2 Riaz JH, Friesen RH. *Anesth. Analg.*, 1979; **58:** 334−336.

Further reading

Hasbury C. *Anaesthesia*, 1982; **37:** 466.
Steward DJ, Izukawa T. *Anesth. Analg.*, 1980; **59:** 81.

Conjoined twins

Siamese twins

Major problems
Two patients
Shared anatomy and physiology
Major surgery
Major blood loss
Overcrowding, confusion

The incidence of this condition is between 1:50000 and
1:200000. Only about 30% of such twins survive the first 24
hours; they are thought to be monozygotic. The way in which
the twins are joined is variable—most commonly they are
joined chest/abdomen to chest/abdomen. However, they may
also be joined back to back, side to side, or head to head. If they
are joined at the pelvis then there may be two, three or four
lower limbs. Sharing of internal organs is a grave complicating
factor.

Important points for the management of these patients are
as follows:

1 There needs to be a multidisciplinary approach to this clinical
problem, with plastic surgeons, orthopaedic, genito-urinary,
general and thoracic surgeons where necessary. There should be
close liaison with the blood bank and all those involved in the
pre-operative evaluation of the situation. The anaesthetists
should be involved at all stages.

2 It is advisable to have two anaesthetists per twin and another
coordinating. Surgery may last many hours.

3 Intensive monitoring with intensive efforts to maintain the
status quo with blood warmers, humidifiers, warming blankets,
fluids, electrolytes, blood, platelets, etc. are all required. To avoid
confusion all tubing going to one twin should be identified by
coloured tape, with all laboratory specimens identified using the
same coloured tape.

4 It has been suggested that with sharing of abdominal organs it
is possible that one twin may suffer adrenal insufficiency—
hydrocortisone is given prophylactically.

5 Should one twin die then skin should be salvaged so as to aid skin cover on the surviving twin, if necessary.

6 It is good practice to have a rehearsal of the roles of the two anaesthetic and surgical teams prior to the actual day of surgery.

7 Minor surgery may be necessary prior to definitive separation.

8 Because of the massive transfusion, use fresh blood if possible.

Further reading

Chao CC, Susetio L, Luu KW, Kwan WF. *Can. Anaesth. Soc. J.*, 1980; **27:** 565–571.

Fournier L, Goulet C, Waugh R, Chouinard R. *Can. Anaesth. Soc. J.*, 1976; **23:** 425–431.

James PD, Lerman J, McLeod ME, Relton JES, Creighton RE. *Can. Anaesth. Soc. J.*, 1985; **32:** 402–411.

Towey RM, Kisia AKL, Jacobacci S, Muoki M. *Anaesthesia,* 1979; **34:** 187–192.

Corpus callosum (agenesis)

Major problems
Ketamine not effective
Associated neurological defects

Agenesis of the corpus callosum is a rare condition which may not be associated with any detectable neurological deficit [1]. The case report describes the use of ketamine in a 3.9 kg child for pneumoencephalography; a total of 50 mg I.M. and 50 mg I.V. were used over a period of 1 hour 45 minutes. Anaesthesia was considered inadequate with bizarre limb movements and eye opening during the procedure. Muscle rigidity led to opisthotonos and breathing became irregular. Diazepam did not help and caused some respiratory depression. There did seem to be some purposeful withdrawal movements during the procedure which suggested that anaesthesia was inadequate.

It is thought that widespread abnormal brain development leads to a reorganisation of the neural pathways which link the cortex and the limbic system. It is this reorganisation which was suggested as the reason for the failure of ketamine to provide adequate anaesthesia.

Reference

1 Russell IF. *Br. J. Anaesth.*, 1979; **51:** 983–985.

Creutzfeldt-Jacob disease

Subacute spongiform encephalopathy

Major problems
Potentially transmissible disease
Autonomic dysfunction

The frequency of this disease is low (2:1 000 000). It appears to be passed on in an autosomal dominant manner but it has also been transmitted from patient to patient and thus it is thought to be a disease caused by an unconventional virus in which the expression of the infection is genetically determined. Dementia, ataxia and diffuse myoclonic jerks are the main components of this disorder. An autonomic abnormality may make the patient unresponsive to atropine and liver function may be compromised.

Transmission of the disease is possible from many body tissues and the incubation period is probably about two and a half years. Great care should be taken to avoid contamination, especially percutaneous contamination. Contaminated skin should be washed (not scrubbed) with a detergent. Open contamination through scratches or needle prick should be managed by cleaning with either a phenolic antiseptic, 0.5% sodium hypochlorite or a 1:3 000 solution of potassium permanganate. Use disposable equipment where possible; non-disposable items should be autoclaved at 121°C (15 p.s.i.) or sterilised using 0.5% solution of sodium hypochlorite, which is also used for cleaning the theatre working area.

Further reading

Gajdusek DC, Gibbs CJ, Asher DM, Brown P, Diwan A, Hoffman P, Nemo G, Rohwer R, White L. *N. Engl. J. Med.*, 1977; **297:** 1253−1258.
MacMurdo SD, Jakymec AJ, Bleyaert AL. *Anesthesiology*, 1984; **60:** 590−592.

Cri du chat

Cat cry syndrome, del (5P) syndrome, 5P
deletion syndrome

Major problems
Possible abnormal larynx and upper airway
Congenital heart disease
Mental and physical retardation

The incidence of this chromosomal disorder (partial deletion of the short arm of chromosome 5) is about 1:50 000. The patients are mentally and physically retarded. The pathognomonic cry is probably of both laryngeal and neurological origins because the larynx is commonly abnormal but not always so. The larynx may be small or narrow and diamond-shaped. Laryngo-malacia may be present and vocal cord paralysis has been reported. The presence of an elongated floppy epiglottis, together with the micro-retrognathia and high arched palate may make tracheal intubation more difficult.

General hypotonia suggests that conservative doses of muscle relaxants should be adequate and the likely presence of congenital heart disease should always be remembered. Respiratory infections are common and may be due to a partially incompetent larynx—postoperative respiratory care may need to be intensive.

Further reading

Yamashita M, Tanioka F, Taniguchi K, Matsuki A, Oyama T. *Anesthesiology,* 1985; **63:** 201–202.

Cushing's syndrome

Major problems
Hypertension
Glucose intolerance and obesity
Osteoporosis
Muscle wasting/electrolyte abnormalities
Neonatal hypoglycaemia

The case reported by Glassford *et al.* [1] was of a patient with Cushing's syndrome undergoing caesarean section. Her blood pressure was 160/100 mmHg, controlled with metoprolol, and she had the classical features which include "moon" facies, malar flush, striae, truncal obesity and thin extremities. The caesarean section was carried out, uneventfully, under epidural anaesthesia.

The common problems associated with Cushing's syndrome are outlined as follows:

1 *Hypercortisolaemia* can cause a retention of sodium and a hyperkalaemic metabolic alkalosis.

2 *Tracheal intubation* can be difficult with the presence of obesity and the "buffalo hump".

3 *Respiratory insufficiency* may result from muscle atrophy and hypokalaemia.

4 *Electrolyte abnormalities* should be corrected before surgery.

5 *Osteoporosis* may cause spinal fractures.

General anaesthesia may be complicated by the hypertensive response to tracheal intubation and spinal anaesthesia may result in catastrophic hypotension. Epidural anaesthesia was considered the technique of choice and the patient intensively monitored using direct measurement of both arterial and central venous pressures.

Costa *et al.* [2] advocated the use of etomidate for the management of patients with Cushing's syndrome—they used 0.02 mg kg^{-1} min^{-1} and noted a peri-operative decrease in cortisol levels that returned to previous levels within eight hours.

References

1 Glassford J, Eagle C, McMorland GH. *Can. Anaesth. Soc. J.*, 1984; **31:** 447–450.
2 Costa J, Ramos D, Massada S, Carvalho D, Pignatelli D. *Anaesthesia*, 1986; **41:** 211–212.

Cystic fibrosis

Major problem
Very limited respiratory reserve

Cystic fibrosis is transmitted as an autosomal recessive trait (1:2500) and results in severe chronic obstructive pulmonary disease. It is a disease of the exocrine glands—those of the gut and respiratory system produce thick secretions and the sweat and parotid glands produce secretions with abnormal electrolyte content. Cough, recurrent pneumonia and chronic air trapping all lead to clinical signs of chronic respiratory disease with bronchiectasis and pulmonary fibrosis. Modern management includes antibiotic therapy, pancreatic enzyme supplements, vitamins and regular effective chest physiotherapy.

The general principles involved in the management of such patients include:

1 Careful pre-operative assessment.

2 Avoidance of respiratory depression thus causing retention of secretions and further atelectasis.

3 Tracheal intubation for all but the most minor procedures so that adequate humidification and effective tracheal toilet are possible.

4 Controlled ventilation—again the aim is to reduce further atelectasis.

5 Appropriate antibiotic therapy.

6 Intensive postoperative physiotherapy with good pain control.

The patient described by Hyde and Harrison[1] had intrathecal morphine (1 mg in 1 ml 0.9% saline—no preservative) for analgesia for childbirth. This was successful and avoided the hazards of hypotension, which would have necessitated a fluid load and the supine position. The spinal injection was carried out with the patient sitting—thus avoiding respiratory embarrassment produced by lying on one side—it was also quicker. Progress of the labour was not affected. This dose of morphine was insufficient to cause respiratory depression and the transient pruritus was treated with intravenous naloxone.

Reference

1 Hyde NH, Harrison DM. *Anesth. Analg.*, 1986; **65:** 1357—1358.

Further reading

Doershuk CF, Reyes AL, Regan AG, Matthews LW. *Anesth. Analg.*, 1972; **51:** 413—421.
Harnik E, Kulzycki L, Gomes MN. *Anesth. Analg.*, 1983; **62:** 357—362.

Cystic hygroma

Major problems
Airway difficulty
Repeated surgery

The vast majority of these fluid-containing lesions are found before two years of age. They can be found elsewhere but the neck is the commonest site; if it occupies the anterior triangle then it may well affect the floor of the mouth. Extension into the chest is possible. The lesions are lymphangiomas and are hamartomatous. Increase in cyst size may occur rapidly—either secondary to infection or due to internal haemorrhage. Complete excision is the treatment of choice but may be difficult if not impossible. Airway involvement is possible with difficulty in eating or drinking leading to a dehydrated, undernourished child. Haemorrhage can be considerable and meticulous haemostasis prior to surgical closure is mandatory.

Cysts impinging on the floor of the mouth or pharynx may need to be aspirated prior to anaesthesia to facilitate airway control—this, however, does make the surgery more difficult. There may be many cysts around the epiglottis and larynx. In addition, local oedema may be present due to compression of venous drainage channels by the hygroma. Great care should be taken during the induction of anaesthesia to avoid total respiratory obstruction. Tracheotomy is difficult in neonates or infants as an elective procedure and much more difficult if required urgently through a cystic swelling. Cystic hygromas do recur and may become infected. Multiple procedures may be necessary.

Further reading

MacDonald DJF. *Anaesthesia*, 1966; **21**: 66–71.
Weller RM. *Anaesthesia*, 1974; **29**: 588–594.

Denervation hypersensitivity

Major problems
Contracture following use of suxamethonium
Hyperkalaemia after suxamethonium

The mechanism of denervation hypersensitivity is uncertain. It is thought that a larger area of the muscle fibre becomes sensitive to acetylcholine, and thus also sensitive to suxamethonium. This results in greater potassium release and a greater abnormal contraction—a contracture (contraction without conduction).

A patient who presented with a brachial plexus lesion was given suxamethonium during an anaesthetic [1]. This resulted in a sustained increase in tone in the affected limb that only relaxed when the remainder of the body was recovering from the effects of the relaxant. This is a common physiological response in many systems to denervation—that is denervation hypersensitivity. Non-depolarising muscle relaxants are preferable as they do not stimulate the motor end plate.

Reference

1 Brim VD. *Br. J. Anaesth.*, 1973; **45:** 222–226.

Dermatomyositis

Polymyositis

Major problems
Muscle weakness
Tendency to pulmonary aspiration
Possible cardiomyopathy

Dermatomyositis is a multisystem disease that presents as muscle weakness associated with a violaceous rash. Immunological mechanisms are thought to be involved in its aetiology; underlying malignancy should always be considered.

The factors of importance to the anaesthetist are the responses to muscle relaxants, the involvement of the muscles of deglutition which may lead to pulmonary aspiration, and the dysrhythmias that accompany the cardiomyopathy, if present. Evidence suggests sensitivity to non-depolarising agents. In one case [1] there was a prolonged response to a normal dose of vecuronium in a patient with polymyositis although no evidence of abnormality of neuromuscular transmission could be found on subsequent EMG assessment. Suxamethonium in another patient [2] produced a short-lived contracture with normal recovery from the block — no fasciculations were seen nor did the serum potassium rise to abnormally high levels. Cricoid pressure is advisable prior to tracheal intubation. These patients need detailed pre-operative assessment and intensive intra-operative monitoring.

References

1 Flusche G, Unger-Sargon J, Lambert DH. *Anesth. Analg.,* 1987; **66**: 188–190.
2 Johns RA, Finholt DA, Stirt JA. *Can. Anaesth. Soc. J.,* 1986; **33**: 71–74.

DiGeorge syndrome

3rd and 4th arch syndrome

Major problems
Hypocalcaemia
Immunological deficiency
Cardiovascular anomalies
Possible airway difficulty

This syndrome results from the failure of correct development of the 3rd and 4th pharyngeal pouches leading to hypoparathyroidism, hypoplasia or absence of the thymus and cardiovascular anomalies which may include vascular rings, tetralogy of Fallot and other aortic abnormalities.

The baby described [1] underwent a thoracotomy for the ligation of a vascular ring that was causing dysphagia. The serum calcium level was stabilised using parenteral calcium and vitamin D. It is important that frequent rapid estimations of the serum calcium can be made. Hyperventilation should be avoided as a low Pa_{CO_2} will result in an alkalosis that may lower the serum calcium. Chelation of calcium by citrated blood is a theoretical possibility should large volumes be given. A fall in calcium is undesirable as cerebral irritability results and the neuromuscular junction becomes more sensitive to depolarising muscle relaxants. Because of the immunological defect, any blood for transfusion should be irradiated to kill off the donor leucocytes and thus prevent a graft versus host reaction. Infection is a potentially grave problem and thus all measures to avoid or combat infection should be taken. The tracheal intubation was slightly difficult because of an underdeveloped mandible. Further problems with the airway may be caused by the vascular abnormalities compressing the trachea—tracheomalacia can result.

Reference

1 Flashburg MH, Dunbar BS, August G, Watson D. *Anesthesiology*, 1983; **58**: 479–481.

Distal muscular dystrophy

Welander muscular atrophy

Major problem

Increased sensitivity to respiratory depressants

This condition is inherited in an autosomal dominant fashion. Initial involvement is confined to the peripheral limb muscles and may slowly spread proximally. It is a benign condition, appearing after the age of 40 years, and although having little effect on life-span can cause considerable disability.

It has been suggested that these patients have an increased sensitivity to thiopentone and other respiratory depressant agents. These should therefore be given carefully. The myocardial muscle may be affected, in which case myocardial depressant agents (including halothane) may result in an exaggerated fall in blood pressure. No problems have been reported with any of the muscle relaxants, although it may be wise to initially administer a reduced dosage and to monitor the effect.

Further reading

Cobham IG, Davis HS. *Anesth. Analg.*, 1964; **43:** 22−29.
Ellis FR. *Br. J. Anaesth.*, 1974; **46:** 603−612.
Wislicki L. *Anaesthesia*, 1962; **17:** 482−487.

Dutch-Kentucky syndrome

Trismus-pseudocamptodactyly

Major problem
Limited mouth opening

This is an autosomal dominant trait which produces marked limitation of mouth opening and a flexion deformity of the fingers when the wrist is extended.

Excision of the coronoid processes enables mouth opening and it was for this procedure that the patient was anaesthetised [1]. Induction of anaesthesia was accomplished with oxygen, nitrous oxide and halothane; a surgeon stood by should an urgent tracheostomy have been necessary. Blind nasal intubation attempts were unsuccessful but intubation was achieved by passing an uncuffed 5.0 mm tube over a flexible paediatric bronchoscope. During this phase of anaesthesia halothane in 100% O_2 was used. Attempts at intubation should not be obsessive to the point where the patient becomes cyanosed.

Reference

1 Browder FH, Lew D, Shahbazian TS. *Anesthesiology,* 1986; **65:** 218−219.

Dwarfism
Skeletal dysplasia with short stature

Major problems
Kyphoscoliosis is common
Some have atlanto-axial instability
Possibility of spinal cord compression
Possibility of congenital heart disease

A division into two broad categories of proportionate and disproportionate is usual, based on external appearance. The different subgroups which fit into these categories are as follows:

Disproportionate
Achondroplasia (see p. 2)
Non-achondroplastic dwarfism (see below)

Proportionate
Mucopolysaccharidoses (see pp. 155–62)
Mucolipidoses
Turner's syndrome (see p. 257)
Others, e.g. familial, endocrine disease, chronic diseases
   Non-achondroplastic dwarfs often have odontoid dysplasia and this in association with atlanto-axial instability can lead to cervical cord compression. Spinal X-rays are essential in dwarfs with neurological symptoms. Cervical flexion can be avoided by a halo head support or similar device.
   The individual features are as follows:

Spondyloepiphyseal dysplasia
(Congenita, tarda and pseudo-achondroplasia.) Kyphoscoliosis, spinal cord compression, and atlanto-occipital instability are common.

Spondylometepiphyseal dysplasia
(see p. 236)

Metaphyseal dysostosis
(Jansen, Schmid, Spahr and cartilage hair hypoplasia.) The spine
is usually normal. There may be abnormalities of the skull in the
Jansen type.

Multiple epiphyseal dysplasia
(Fairbank's disease.) Usually no problems.

Chondroectodermal dysplasia
(Ellis-van-Creveld syndrome.) The patients usually have a single
atrium and small defective teeth.

Diastrophic dwarfism
Cleft palate and scoliosis are common.

Metatropic dwarfism
These patients have progressive scoliosis.

Silver syndrome
Disproportionately large head with narrow mouth and micrognathia (difficult intubation). Café au lait patches on the skin.

Further reading

Walts LF, Finerman G, Wyatt GM. *Can. Anaesth. Soc. J.*, 1975; **22:** 703−709.

Dysautonomia
Familial dysautonomia (Riley-Day syndrome),
idiopathic autonomic dysfunction, secondary dysautonomia

Major problems
Cardiovascular instability
Respiratory control disturbances
Denervation sensitivity

Familial dysautonomia

This is an autosomal recessive condition that causes a reduction in the number of sensory and sympathetic neurones. It presents in childhood. There is poor perception of pain and temperature, muscular tone is abnormal leading to scoliosis, postural hypotension occurs and there is an insensitivity to hypercarbia and hypoxia. Chronic chest infection is common as a result of recurrent aspiration associated with feeding difficulties.

Controlled ventilation is mandatory and respiration should be carefully assessed postoperatively. Blood pressure should be monitored closely and any fluid or blood loss replaced quickly. These patients are unable to produce a sympathetic response— noradrenaline availability is reduced by 60%. It is not certain whether there is a reduction in synthesis or a failure to release what noradrenaline is available. Because of the chronic exposure to low levels of catecholamines there is a supersensitivity to exogenous transmitter agents (both adrenergic and cholinergic). Inotropic agents should be used with great care.

Different authors state different preferences for inhalational agents/muscle relaxants/cardiovascular support drugs. It would appear that the response to neuromuscular blocking agents is normal and by their use inhalational agents that are likely to depress both the myocardium and vasculature can be avoided. Anticholinesterases should be used in very conservative doses because of the denervation sensitivity.

Idiopathic autonomic dysfunction (IAD)

This condition appears in the middle years of life and is associated with gross cardiovascular instability—an inadequate baroreceptor reflex together with a fixed heart rate can lead to the most profound falls in blood pressure on induction of anaesthesia where respiratory assistance is required and thus the thoracic pump mechanism is lost and replaced by a Valsalva manoeuvre.

Pre-operative preparation may limit the extent to which the blood pressure falls—the patient should sleep with a 25° head-up tilt, a technique which is called 'postural training'. Pre-operative treatment with 9 alpha-fludrocortisone is also effective because this increases the blood volume, and may in the long term increase peripheral resistance. Prior to induction of anaesthesia elastic stockings should be applied to the legs to prevent venous pooling and a large bore cannula inserted into a vein. Pre-loading with fluid may be desirable. Elevated legs will also minimise acute changes. Blood pressure should be measured directly and, ideally, consideration should be given to central venous pressure and pulmonary artery wedge pressure measurement.

Secondary dysautonomia

Autonomic dysfunction due to a disease process that affects neuronal transmission is possible and thus a similar picture to IAD may be found in such disease processes. Diabetes mellitus is the commonest. The problems and precautions are similar to those found in IAD.

Further reading

Familial dysautonomia
Cox RG, Sumner E. *Anaesthesia*, 1983; **38**: 293.
Inkster JS. *Br. J. Anaesth.*, 1971; **43**: 509—512.
McCaughey TJ. *Can. Anaesth. Soc. J.*, 1965; **12**: 558—568.
Meridy HW, Creighton RE. *Can. Anaesth. Soc. J.*, 1971; **18**: 563—570.
Stenqvist O, Sigurdsson J. *Anaesthesia*, 1982; **37**: 929—932.

Idiopathic autonomic dysfunction
Hutchinson RC. *Anaesthesia*, 1986; **41**: 663.
Sweeney BP, Jones S, Langford RM. *Anaesthesia*, 1985; **40**: 783—786.

Ebstein's anomaly

Major problems
Cyanosis, dyspnoea, congestive cardiac failure
Right to left shunt—parodoxical emboli
Enlarged venous pool

Ebstein's anomaly involves the migration of part of the tricuspid valve into the right ventricle so that the right atrium is enlarged and part of its wall is ventricular. There are associated dysrhythmias and possibly an atrial septal defect. The pulmonary vascular resistance may be increased and a right to left shunt occurs. Symptomatology is very variable, from nothing to severe disablement. All such patients should have antibiotic cover to protect them against bacterial endocarditis.

Systemic vascular resistance should be maintained in an attempt to maintain the status quo and not make the shunt worse. To combat hypotension agents with alpha adrenergic agonist activity are the best; phenylephrine or metaraminol are recommended. These potent drugs may have adverse effects on uterine blood flow during pregnancy. During pregnancy there is an increased risk of cardiac failure—if an epidural local anaesthetic block is considered suitable then binding of the legs with crepe bandage, fluid loading (with care) and a two catheter technique (to minimise local anaesthetic dose and cardiovascular effects) is suggested. Syntocinon is preferable to ergometrine because it increases the pulmonary vascular resistance. Central venous lines should not be allowed to migrate into the right atrium as dysrhythmias may be initiated.

An unusual side effect, which results from a grossly enlarged right atrium, is the ineffectiveness of a bolus of hypnotic agent. The bolus becomes markedly diluted in the large venous pool and does not reach a concentration where consciousness is lost. Hypotension may occur with the larger doses required. Elsten's patient [1] had a right atrium of 5 litres capacity.

Reference

1 Elsten JL, Kim YD, Hanowell ST, Macnamara TE. *Anesth. Analg.*, 1981; **60:** 909–910.

Further reading

Bengtsson IM, Magno R, Wickstrom I. *Br. J. Anaesth.*, 1977; **49:** 501–503.
Halpern S, Gidwaney A, Gates B. *Can. Anaesth. Soc. J.*, 1983; **32:** 244–247.
Linter SPK, Clarke K. *Br. J. Anaesth.*, 1984; **56:** 203–205.

Ehlers-Danlos syndrome

Major problems
Bleeding diathesis
Fragile skin and tissues

This is a connective tissue disorder which is inherited in an autosomal dominant manner. In most patients the clinical findings and the symptomatology are minimal. However, the patients with the severe manifestations of the disease are at great risk—principally from haemorrhage. Coagulation studies are normal and the defect is probably in the capillary wall. The syndrome also involves skin, which tears easily and heals leaving 'cigarette paper' scars, and hypermobility of the joints. This may lead to chronic subluxation. Mitral valve prolapse/regurgitation, conduction defects, pneumothoraces, and dilatation of the gastrointestinal tract and trachea are all seen frequently in the Ehlers-Danlos syndrome.

Avoid intramuscular injections, avoid unnecessary vessel cannulation (particularly occult sites like the internal jugular or subclavian veins) and avoid regional anaesthesia. However, the patients described by Abouleish [1] had regional anaesthesia (caudal, epidural and subarachnoid) without ill effect—they appear not to have had the severe ecchymotic form of the disease. Be gentle when handling, moving and positioning these patients.

Reference

1 Abouleish E. *Br. J. Anaesth.*, 1980; **52:** 1283−1286.

Further reading

Dolan P, Sisko F, Riley E. *Anesthesiology*, 1980; **52:** 266−269.

Eisenmenger syndrome

Major problems
Intolerance of systemic hypotension
Paradoxical air embolism
Bacterial endocarditis
Polycythaemia and thromboembolism
Reduced uptake of inhaled agents

Eisenmenger syndrome includes any condition in which there is a communication between pulmonary and systemic circulation resulting in pulmonary vascular disease of such severity that right-to-left shunting occurs. The communication between the pulmonary and systemic circulation may be at the aorto-pulmonary level, at atrial level or at ventricular level. Patients may develop the reversed shunt when very young or may live for decades before this adverse change occurs. When it does occur it may progress rapidly. High blood flow through the defect (left to right) probably initiates the events that lead to changes in the pulmonary vascular bed and pulmonary hypertension. This inexorably results in a change in the haemodynamics (a bi-directional or right-to-left shunt) and hypoxia.

The anaesthetists' aim must be to avoid increasing the shunt from right-to-left and thus avoid producing a vicious circle of hypoxia, myocardial depression, hypotension, increased shunt, hypoxia....

The following recommendations should be considered:

1 Minimise any fall in systemic vascular resistance. Use ketamine, for example, and have an alpha-agonist at hand. Alternatively, give prophylactic metaraminol (1 mg intravenously), methoxamine, or phenylephrine. Monitor the arterial pressure directly.

2 Maintain myocardial contractility—avoid myocardial depressants and bradycardia and maintain venous return.

3 Maintain adequate oxygenation in an attempt to offset the hypoxia due to the shunt.

4 Respond quickly and adequately to fluid loss. Polycythaemia may exist; crystalloid and colloid should be used initially to replace blood loss. Intravascular thrombosis is possible and is a major hazard of using pulmonary flotation catheters and central venous lines. This form of monitoring should be carefully considered in patients with Eisenmenger syndrome as they have proved fatal.

5 Mortality is high—almost 30% in pregnancy. Caesarean section should be avoided if possible as vaginal delivery is safer and may be conducted under epidural analgesia to facilitate instrumentation if necessary. Continuous lumbar epidural anaesthesia has been used for lower abdominal surgery but the systemic blood pressure must be maintained.

Further reading

Asling JH, Fung DL. *Anesth. Analg.*, 1974; **53**: 965–968.
Crawford JS, Mills WG, Pentecost BL. *Br. J. Anaesth.*, 1971; **43**: 1091–1094.
Devitt JH, Noble WH, Byrick RJ. *Anesthesiology*, 1982; **57**: 335–337.
Foster JMG, Jones RM. *Ann. R. Coll. Surg. (Eng.)*, 1984; **66**: 353–355.
Lumley J, Whitwam JG, Morgan M. *Anesth. Analg.*, 1977; **56**: 543–547.

Engelmann's disease

Camarati-Engelmann disease,
osteopathia hyperostotica sclerotisans multiplex infantalis

Major problems
Airway difficulty
Limited mouth opening
Limited neck mobility

This is a very rare disease of the skeleton. It is a form of osteo-petrosis (marble bone disease), a generalised form of diaphyseal dysplasia. It is dominantly inherited. Frontal bossing, deafness, blindness and hyperostosis leading to generalised skeletal abnormalities may all be present.

The patient described [1] proved to be an intubation problem which was overcome by a modified Waters technique—retro-grade passage of a ureteric stillette through the cricothyroid membrane and vocal cords, and thence through the nose to guide the passage of a naso-tracheal tube.

Reference

1 Mason J, Slee I. *Anaesthesia,* 1968; **23:** 250—252.

Eosinophilic myositis

Major problems
None

This is a rare inflammatory myopathy; it may be idiopathic or secondary to parasitic infestation. The patient described [1] did not prove to be a difficult anaesthetic problem—the action of atracurium was marginally prolonged. Agents that may have triggered malignant hyperpyrexia were avoided.

The hypereosinophilic syndrome (a severe generalised eosinophilia) is more hazardous—hepatosplenomegaly and congestive heart failure due to a restrictive cardiomyopathy may make anaesthesia difficult. These patients may be on steroids or cytotoxic agents.

Reference

1 Farag HM, Naguib M. Gyani H, Ibrahim AW. *Anesth. Analg.,* 1986; **65:** 903−904.

Epidermolysis bullosa

Epidermolysis bullosa dystrophica

Major problems
Scarred skin and mouth
Airway difficulty
Very delicate skin and oral mucosa
Hypoproteinaemia
Anaemia and general debility

Epidermolysis bullosa (EB) is the common name for a group of skin conditions of varying severity, of various modes of inheritance and in which the common pathological feature is that of blister formation in response to friction and trauma. There are two main categories—scarring and non-scarring.

Non-scarring
Generalised EB simplex (Koebner)
Localised EB simplex (Weber-Cockayne)
Junctional EB*†

Scarring
Dominant dystrophic EB*
Recessive dystrophic EB*†
Acquired EB

The formation of blisters is associated with protein loss, infection (beta haemolytic streptococcus) and possibly haemorrhage. Scarring of the raw area is the chronic insult to the acute problem. Digits become mutilated and the mouth and oesophagus strictured.

The tongue may be completely immobilised and this, together with dysplastic teeth, may cause tracheal intubation to be difficult. An oropharyngeal airway is not usually necessary or desir-

*Either moderately or severely debilitating.
†Perioral, oral and airway involvement to be expected.

74

able. It is not necessary because the tongue is fixed anteriorly to the mandible and cannot fall back into the pharynx, and it is undesirable because of possible trauma to the palate and pharynx. It has been repeatedly noted that the larynx and trachea do not seem to produce blisters in response to intubation —this may be because the mucosa is ciliated columnar and not squamous. Tracheal intubation should not be regarded as hazardous as long as the mouth and pharynx are not traumatised. A Macintosh laryngoscope is preferred to a Magill laryngoscope because the former avoids contact with the posterior aspect of the epiglottis and thus diminishes the likelihood of supraglottic obstruction by an epiglottic blister. A pre-warmed, soft, plastic endotracheal tube is preferred and it should be well-lubricated. Adhesive strapping should not be used at all and the tube should be gently tied in place. The cuff should be inflated sufficiently to just stop any air leak, as always. Two patients are reported to have developed spontaneous laryngeal stenosis.

If a mask is used, the face should be protected with paraffin gauze impregnated with hydrocortisone cream. Similar treatment should be used under the chin where fingers commonly leave their imprints when holding a mask. The eyes should similarly be well protected. Other measures to minimise skin trauma include the stitching in of intravenous cannula and protecting the cannula with wadding and crepe bandage. Non-adhesive ECG electrodes and diathermy plates are best. The skin under the blood pressure cuff should also be protected by a thin layer of wadding.

Views on the use of regional techniques are varied but Broster [1] provided anaesthesia for caesarean section by using subarachnoid and epidural block without incident.

Steroids are now infrequently used but the patient may be taking phenytoin. This is used to reduce the activity of the collagenase that appears to be responsible for the blister formation. Should bleeding from a blister site occur then a swab soaked in 1:200 000 ephedrine should be applied. The patient should be screened for porphyria as reports have suggested an association with epidermolysis bullosa. This association has however been questioned [2].

References

1 Broster T, Placek R, Eggers GWN. *Anesth. Analg.*, 1987; **66:** 341−343.
2 Spargo PM, Smith GB. *Anesth. Analg.*, 1988; **67:** 297−298.

Further reading

James I, Wark H. *Anesthesiology*, 1982; **56:** 323−326.
Holzman RS, Worthen HM, Johnson KL. *Can. Anaesth. Soc. J.*, 1987; **34:** 395−399.
Idvall J. *Acta Anaesthesiol. Scand.*, 1987; **31:** 658−660.
Tomlinson AA. *Anaesthesia*, 1983; **38:** 485−491.

Erythema multiforme

Stevens Johnson syndrome

Major problems
Delicate skin and mucous membranes
Airway difficulties
Increased susceptibility to secondary infection

Painful skin eruptions develop which progress to bullae, erosions and ulcers. These may occur in any site, but in particular affect the mouth and face. When the eyes and genitalia are additionally affected this becomes the Stevens Johnson syndrome. The aetiology is unclear, predisposing factors including acute bacterial or viral infections, drug idiosyncracy and underlying malignancy. It may affect any age group, but is more common in children.

The mucous membranes and affected area of skin are especially delicate. Minor trauma may result in painful blisters and erosions. Monitoring should therefore be attached carefully, e.g. use non-adhesive ECG electrodes and padding under the sphygmomanometer cuff. It is best to avoid all instrumentation of the mouth, including intubation, airways, facemasks and nasogastric tube. If this is necessary plenty of lubricant should be used and the patient treated very gently. The patients are prone to infection and so strict asepsis is necessary with all procedures, including intravenous access. Intermittent ketamine has been successfully used for anaesthesia in patients with this disorder [1]. The pleura may be affected by bullae formation, leading to pleural effusion or pneumothorax. Myocarditis may be present. It is therefore important to assess cardiac and respiratory reserve before considering anaesthesia in these patients.

Reference

1 Cucchiara RF, Dawson B. *Anesthesiology*, 1971; **35**: 537–539.

Exomphalos

Major problems
Heat loss
Respiratory failure
Infection
Other congenital abnormalities

During early fetal development the gut outgrows the abdominal cavity. Failure of the gut, and possibly other abdominal organs, to be re-accommodated by the abdomen later on results in exomphalos. It occurs once in 10 000 live births. The exomphalos may or may not be covered in peritoneum because rupture of the peritoneal membrane may occur during delivery or afterwards.

Half of these babies have other congenital abnormalities. The babies should be nursed in an incubator, the stomach should be aspirated regularly by a nasogastric tube and fluids administered intravenously. A paralytic ileus is common postoperatively and thus reliable venous access is mandatory for some time, perhaps weeks. Elective postoperative ventilation is advisable as respiratory embarrassment is certain. Mortality is high, almost 50%. A quarter of the deaths were associated with the other congenital abnormalities, infection with another third and respiratory failure was implicated in over half.

Further reading

Ryan DW. *Anaesthesia*, 1973; **28**: 407–414.

Facial diplegia (congenital)

Moebius syndrome, Mobius syndrome

Major problems
Weak cough reflex
Weak gag reflex

This rare congenital abnormality of the cranial nerves may produce either complete or partial facial paralysis. The patient's facial appearance is therefore expressionless and "mask-like". It is inherited in an autosomal dominant fashion and the patient would be expected to have a normal life span. Cranial nerves 6 and 7 are the most commonly affected, although others may occasionally be involved, leading to weakness or paralysis of the palate or tongue. The result is that the patient may have difficulties in chewing, swallowing and coughing.

The weakness in the muscles controlling the face and upper airway results in repeated minor episodes of tracheal aspiration leading, eventually, to chronic respiratory problems. The patient's respiratory status should therefore be carefully assessed pre-operatively. Respiratory difficulties may be encountered in the postoperative period and it may be advisable to leave the tracheal tube *in situ* until the patient is fully awake. An association with micrognathia has been suggested and if this is present intubation difficulties may be experienced.

Further reading

Krajcirik WJ, Azar I, Opperman S, Lear E. *Anesth. Analg.*, 1985; **64:** 371–372.

Familial periodic paralysis

Major problems
Muscle weakness
Hypo/hyperkalaemia

The major symptom of this condition is skeletal muscle weakness of such a degree that respiratory support may be necessary. Hypokalaemia, hyperkalaemia or normokalaemia have all been reported during the attacks. Transmission of the disease is considered to be autosomal dominant, predominantly in males, worse in childhood and precipitated by high carbohydrate intake, excitement, trauma, cold, infection and menstruation. It is associated with adrenal and thyroid tumours. Only patients with the hypokalaemic variety are reported in the anaesthetic literature.

To reduce patient stress the anaesthetist should counsel the patient and, if necessary, prescribe an anxiolytic agent. Concentrated dextrose infusions should be avoided, sodium restricted and potassium supplemented by the addition of $2 \, g l^{-1}$ of potassium chloride to infused fluids. The patient should not be allowed to become cold and the ECG should be closely monitored.

Siler and Discavage [1] used suxamethonium without adverse reaction, Horton [2] used no relaxant but monitored neuromuscular transmission and Fozard [3] avoided muscle relaxants also. Volatile agents that produce muscular relaxation should be used with caution—a neuroleptanalgesia technique or regional local anaesthetic block should be considered. Monitor the patient closely in the postoperative period for incipient weakness.

References

1 Siler JN, Discavage WJ. *Anesthesiology*, 1975; **43:** 489–490.
2 Horton B. *Anesthesiology*, 1977; **47:** 308–310.
3 Fozard JR. *Anaesthesia*, 1983; **38:** 293–294.

Fanconi syndrome

Lignac-Fanconi syndrome, renal tubular acidosis,
cystinosis, de Toni Fanconi syndrome

Major problem
Large fluid and electrolyte changes leading to
muscle weakness and acidosis

The proximal renal tubule dysfunction results in hyperamino-
aciduria, glycosuria and hyperphosphaturia. Potassium, bicarbonate and water are also lost. This syndrome may be inherited
(autosomal recessive, 1:40 000) or acquired. The acquired form is
associated with amyloidosis, cystinosis, galactosaemia, myeloma,
toxins and Wilson's disease. Patients are of short stature with
osteomalacia.

Polyuria may lead to hypovolaemia which, with a reduction in
tissue perfusion, may exacerbate the acidosis. Circulating volume
should be continuously assessed by central venous pressure
measurement (minimal requirement). Urine output should be
continuously monitored as should the potassium concentration
and acid base status. Pre-emptive bicarbonate administration is
advisable. The biochemical derangements of patients with the
Fanconi syndrome differ and thus the individual's electrolyte
status should be carefully studied.

Further reading

Joel M, Rosales JK. *Anesthesiology*, 1981; **55**: 455−456.

Fetal alcohol syndrome

Major problems
Airway difficulty
Cardiac abnormalities

This is a condition resulting from the teratogenic effects of alcohol. The incidence is reported to be 1−2:1000, with other reports of partial expression of the disorder up to 5:1000. Features present in more than 80% of patients are mental retardation, microcephaly, irritability, smallness for age, short palpebral fissures, retrognathia in infancy. A hyperplastic maxilla is found in over half the patients. Murmurs are found frequently—usually an atrial or ventricular septal defect. Hernias and squints are also common.

The two patients described by Finucane [1] were both extremely difficult to intubate. In one, tracheal intubation was abandoned and the hernias repaired using a mask and airway technique—with difficulty.

Reference

1 Finucane BT. *Can. Anaesth. Soc. J.*, 1980; **27:** 574−575.

Freeman-Sheldon syndrome

Windmill-vane-hand syndrome, cranio-carpo-tarsal dysplasia,
whistling face syndrome

Major problems
Airway difficulty
Myopathy
Vascular access

This craniofacial-dysotosis is inherited in an autosomal dominant
manner; it has been suggested that it is the muscular abnormality that causes the craniofacial deformity. Contracture of the
facial, pharyngeal and anterior neck muscles contributes to the
intubation difficulties—pursed mouth, small mandible, high
arched palate, short neck and a high larynx.

The myopathy can lead to kyphoscoliosis and the chronic
upper airway obstruction to pulmonary hypertension. There are
many associated problems—feeding difficulties, spina bifida
occulta, inguinal herniae, and forearm and lower limb orthopaedic abnormalities. Cardiac defects and mental retardation are
not included. Vascular access may be difficult due to a thickening
of subcutaneous tissues and plaster casts. Malignant hyperpyrexia has not been reported with this myopathy.

Further reading

Laishley RS, Roy WL. *Can. Anaesth. Soc. J.*, 1986; **33**: 388–393.

Friedreich's ataxia

Major problems
Heart failure
Respiratory insufficiency
Muscle weakness
Kyphoscoliosis

This is the commonest of the inherited ataxias; it is transmitted in an autosomal recessive manner. Progressive degeneration of the spinocerebellar and pyramidal tracts, together with atrophy of the dorsal root ganglion, produces a mixed upper and lower motor neurone picture—some writers have likened it to amyotrophic lateral sclerosis. It has been postulated that the kidney is unable to retain taurine and this upsets the biochemistry involved in lipoprotein synthesis and also disrupts pyruvate, bilirubin and calcium metabolism.

The factors of importance to the anaesthetist are the cardiomyopathy that may easily lead to heart failure, the muscle weakness that leads to kyphoscoliosis, the restrictive lung function and the possible abnormal response to muscle relaxants. Neither Bell *et al.* [1], nor Bird and Strunin [2], found abnormal duration of action of non-depolarisers (atracurium, d-tubocurarine or pancuronium) but recommend neuromuscular transmission monitoring. Suxamethonium was not used but a hyperkalaemic response would not be anticipated—electromyography is normal.

For the production of hypotension nitroprusside proved a problem (resistant tachycardia) but isoflurane was satisfactory. If cardiomyopathy does exist then intensive cardiovascular monitoring is warranted. Diabetes mellitus is associated with this condition.

References

1 Bell CF, Kelly JM, Jones RS. *Anaesthesia,* 1986; **41:** 296−301.
2 Bird TM, Strunin L. *Anesthesiology,* 1984; **60:** 377−380.

Fructose-1,6-diphosphatase deficiency

Major problems
Hypoglycaemia
Metabolic acidosis

Fructose-1,6-diphosphatase deficiency is rare. The liver cannot produce glucose from fructose, lactate, glycerol or alanine, thus once liver glycogen stores are depleted hypoglycaemia results with lactic acidosis. The enzyme deficiency also causes the accumulation of fructose-1,6-diphosphate which leads to pyruvate production and more lactic acid.

The precautions to be taken include the total avoidance of fructose, which induces hypoglycaemia, for 24−48 hours preoperatively, and the infusion of sufficient glucose during this period of fasting. Frequent measurements of blood glucose and the acid-base status should be made. During lactic acidosis do not use lactated Ringer's (Hartmann's) solution. Sorbitol should not be given as it is converted to fructose. Sodium bicarbonate should be used to treat the metabolic acidosis.

Further reading

Hashimoto Y, Watanabe H, Satou M. *Anesth. Analg.*, 1978; **57**: 503−506.

Fused jaws

Major problem
Airway difficulty

Fusion of the jaws is a very rare abnormality and is associated with cleft palate, aglossia, facial hemiatrophy and retrognathia.

A nasogastric tube should be passed to enable feeding and pre-operative aspiration of gastric contents. Blind nasal intubation is not advised—the trauma may compromise the airway further. Should total loss of airway control occur then a tracheostomy would be required. A variety of agents (ketamine, gamma-hydroxybutyrate, ether, lignocaine) were used by the different authors in an attempt to maintain laryngeal competence or to suppress it to enable intubation. Seraj et al. [1] used one nostril for insufflation of anaesthetic gases whilst the other was reserved for pharyngeal suction. Alfery et al. [2] used a fibreoptic bronchoscope (3.2 mm) to visualise the larynx through one nostril and passed the endotracheal tube down the other. Together with intravenous sedation and head and neck manipulation the trachea was successfully intubated.

References

1 Seraj MA, Yousif M, Channa AB. *Anaesthesia,* 1984; **39**: 695−698.
2 Alfery DD, Ward CF, Harwood IR, Mannino FL. *Anesthesiology,* 1979; **51**: 340−342.

Further reading

Brown TCK, Dwyer ME. *Anaesthesia,* 1985; **40**: 597−598.

Gardner's syndrome

Major problems
Intestinal malignancy with haemorrhage
Airway difficulty

This is a dominantly inherited condition which presents with intestinal polyposis, multiple fibrous tissue tumours and osteomas. Although the intestinal polyps are premalignant the other tumours are histologically benign.

The patient described [1] had repeated surgery for recurrent fibromas in her neck, their growth increased rapidly when she became pregnant and caused dysphagia and dyspnoea. Airway obstruction increased and necessitated anaesthetic/surgical intervention. A tracheostomy was made but was subsequently allowed to close; in retrospect this was probably a mistake.

Reference

1 Pappas MT, Katz J, Finestone SC. *Anesth. Analg.*, 1971; **50**: 340–343.

Gastroparesis (diabetic)

Major problem
Pulmonary aspiration of gastric contents

"Any diabetics with diffuse symmetrical peripheral neuropathy may have autonomic neuropathy as well" [1]. If they have an autonomic neuropathy then they have a 30% chance of having delayed gastric emptying. The patient should be asked about gastric symptoms—post-prandial fullness or inability to eat a large meal.

Metoclopramide and domperidone have been found to be effective in improving gastric emptying and thus should be used prophylactically. More active measures may be deemed necessary, depending on the circumstances, to empty the stomach. Airway protection with cricoid pressure and tracheal intubation are absolute requirements.

Reference

1 Mulhall BP, O'Fearghail M. *Anaesthesia,* 1984; **39:** 468—469.

Glomus jugulare

Chemodectoma, non-chromaffin paraganglionoma,
receptoma

Major problems
Long duration of surgery
Haemorrhage
CNS protection

These tumours arise from paraganglia found around the jugular
bulb in the temporal bone. They are histologically benign but
spread to involve vessels, nerves and bone both intra- and extra-
cranial. They are highly vascular, sometimes arising from the
carotid bodies or the cervical sympathetic chain, and normally
non-secreting although some do release catecholamines [1].

Surgery is the definitive treatment and involves painstaking
dissection within the neck and temporal bone; Mather and
Webster [2] recommend a two-stage approach to limit the opera-
tion length on each occasion to about 10 hours. The second half
was carried out one week after the first. Moderate hypotension
was used. Braude *et al.* [3] used surface induced hypothermia
with normocarbia to facilitate the intracranial excision of the
tumour extension—steroids, barbiturates and mannitol were also
used to protect the brain following the ligation of the internal
carotid artery. Blood pressure was maintained at almost normal
levels to ensure cerebral perfusion and adequate cross circulation.

Most of these tumours are not secretory but the patient described by Clarke *et al.* [1] had a catecholamine secreting mass
and was managed like a phaeochromocytoma. The patient was
pretreated with phenoxybenzamine to provide alpha-blockade
and with propranolol for beta-blockade. A neuroleptic technique
was used for anaesthesia with phentolamine and nitroprusside
administration as required. Hypothermia to 31°C was used to
enable the excision of the tumour.

Glomus jugulare

References

1 Clarke AD, Matheson H, Boddie HG. *Anaesthesia*, 1976; **31:** 1225−1230.
2 Mather SP, Webster NR. *Anaesthesia*, 1986; **41:** 856−860.
3 Braude BM, Hockman R, McIntosh WA, Hagen D. *Anaesthesia*, 1986; **41:** 861−865.

Glossopharyngeal neuralgia

Major problems
Bradycardia
Asystole
Convulsions

On stimulation of the glossopharyngeal nerve, the glossopharyn-geal—vagal reflex arc causes bradycardia or asystole. Cerebral hypoxia resulting from the syncope may produce convulsions.

In the patient described [1], an invasive tumour caused the glosso-pharyngeal neuralgia which was not relieved by local anaesthetic topically applied to the tonsillar bed. The reflex was only broken when the 'arc' was disrupted surgically at cranio-tomy. Transvenous pacing was used to maintain the heart rate. However, even a normal heart rate may not maintain the blood pressure—a noradrenaline infusion was available. The mechanism behind the hypotension occurring, in the presence of a normal heart rate, with the reflex is unclear but the patient may have been on the verge of hypovolaemia. Lesions anywhere along the route of the glossopharyngeal nerve may cause the reflex to be evoked.

Reference

1 Roa NL, Krupin BR. *Anesthesiology*, 1981; **54:** 426—428.

Glucagonoma

Major problems
None

Tumours of the alpha cells of the islets of Langerhans in the pancreas are rare. These cells normally secrete glucagon which has hyperglycaemic and inotropic properties. To diagnose the syndrome of glucagonoma is difficult; a skin rash (necrolytic migratory erythema), glucose intolerance and hypoamino-acidaemia may be present. The demonstration of a tumour mass and elevated glucagon levels, together with hyperglycaemia, are mandatory.

Nicoll [1] found no overt physiological response to the surgical manipulation of the tumour. Even though glucagon concentration rose dramatically it did not reach pharmacologically active levels. Anaesthesia was unremarkable—diazepam premedication, fentanyl, thiopentone, alcuronium, nitrous oxide, oxygen and halothane. Dextrose solutions were avoided.

Reference

1 Nicoll JMV, Catling SJ. *Anaesthesia*, 1985; **40:** 152–157.

Glucose 6-phosphate dehydrogenase deficiency

Favism

Major problem
Haemolysis

Patients with G6PD deficiency are unable to increase the rate of oxidation of glucose in the presence of oxidative agents and thus oxidation of cell proteins occurs. The oxidation of haemoglobin forms methaemoglobin and oxidation of cell membranes causes haemolysis. The inheritance is sex-linked and the highest incidence (35%) is found in Sardinians and Sephardic Jews. Negroes have an incidence of 13% and Caucasians 1−3%. There are many varieties of this condition.

Drugs to avoid, because of their haemolytic tendency, include aspirin, methylene blue, probenecid, vitamin K, chloramphenicol and quinidine. The ingestion of Fava beans (broad beans) also causes haemolysis, hence the alternative name Favism. Isosorbide dinitrate, prilocaine and sodium nitroprusside should also be avoided. This list is *not* exhaustive. Anaemia, jaundice, splenic enlargement and loin pain are all possible following haemolysis. Renal failure may occur. It should always be included in the differential diagnosis of postoperative jaundice.

Further reading

Gilbertson AA, Boulton TB. *Anaesthesia*, 1967; **22:** 607−630.
Shapley JM, Wilson JR. *Can. Anaesth. Soc. J.*, 1973; **20:** 390−392.
Smith CL, Snowdon SL. *Anaesthesia*, 1987; **42:** 281−288.

Glycogen storage disease I

Von Gierke's disease, glucose 6-phosphatase deficiency

Major problems
Hypoglycaemia
Metabolic acidosis
Bleeding diathesis

In this condition there is an inability to produce glucose from glycogen and thus hypoglycaemia, ketosis and increased gluconeogenesis occurs. Maintenance therapy includes regular feeding and oral alkali. Growth and development are retarded. It is transmitted in an autosomal recessive manner and primarily affects the liver and kidneys.

The hypoglycaemia must be controlled—if not by regular feeding, by nasogastric infusions; if not by the enteral route then intravenously. Correction of the biochemistry corrects the bleeding diathesis which is due to a platelet dysfunction. Total parenteral nutrition may be necessary, or portacaval shunt formation to prevent the persistence of hyperlipidaemia, hyperuricaemia and growth retardation.

The aim during surgery must be to maintain blood glucose levels and treat metabolic acidosis if it occurs. Hyperventilation should be avoided; during respiratory alkalosis lactate is liberated from muscle but these patients cannot adequately metabolise it, thus acidosis is increased. Lactated physiological solutions should also be avoided.

Further reading

Bevan JC. *Anaesthesia,* 1980; **35:** 699–702.
Cox JM. *Anesthesiology,* 1968; **29:** 1221–1225.
Casson H. *Br. J. Anaesth.,* 1975; **47:** 969–975.

Glycogen storage disease II

Acid maltase deficiency, Pompe's disease,
alpha-1,4-glucosidase deficiency

Major problems
Heart failure
Skeletal muscle weakness
Hypoxia

In this glycogen storage disease there is a deposition of glycogen throughout the body. It is inherited in an autosomal recessive manner and is rare. The enzyme deficiency is found in the lysosomes not in the cytoplasm and blood sugar is therefore normal. The baby becomes floppy and develops cardiomegaly; air hunger may be present due to bronchial compression by the enlarged heart. Death usually occurs before the age of one year. Bone marrow transplantation may offer some hope for these patients.

Drugs used to induce anaesthesia must not make the cardiac failure worse—some of these patients have 'congestive' cardiac failure whilst others have an 'obstructive' outflow picture. McFarlane and Soni [1] debate the issue about choice of agents but recommend the agent that is familiar and monitor the patient closely. The myopathy associated with the condition may make muscle relaxants unnecessary, but should relaxation be required vecuronium is recommended. It provides cardiovascular stability and its elimination by the liver is unaffected by the disease. Suxamethonium is contraindicated because muscle damage occurs, secondary to the rupture of lysosomes, and there is the risk of potassium leak together with the remote possibility of malignant hyperpyrexia. The muscle weakness may cause the patient to require postoperative respiratory support. Hypoxia is a problem and may be due to aspiration pneumonia, lower conductive airway obstruction or due to macroglossia; a 'pseudo-macroglossia' may be present due to the protrusion of the tongue during air hunger.

A caudal block has been suggested as suitable for some surgery and is a relatively trouble-free technique. Rosen and Broadman [2] used the inguinal paravascular "3 in 1" block to facilitate muscle biopsy. It was performed under sedation with ketamine. They argued that there was always the potential danger of dural puncture and high spinal anaesthesia with a caudal block. These patients carry a high risk during anaesthesia—monitor them well.

References

1 McFarlane HJ, Soni N. *Anaesthesia,* 1986; **41:** 1219−1224.
2 Rosen KR, Broadman LM. *Can. Anaesth. Soc. J.,* 1986; **33:** 790.

Further reading

Cox JM. *Anesthesiology,* 1968; **29:** 1221−1225.
Kaplan R. *Anesthesiology Review;* 1986; **7:** 21−28.

Glycogen storage disease V
Muscle glycogen phosphorylase deficiency, McArdle's disease

Major problems
Muscle fatigue
Myoglobinuria (avoid suxamethonium)

The absence of muscle glycogen phosphorylase, transmitted in an autosomal recessive manner, leads to the accumulation of glycogen in muscle and lack of lactate during ischaemic exercise. On exertion the muscle becomes painful, stiff and is easily fatigued. Myoglobinuria occurs and has occasionally caused renal failure. Whilst living within their exercise tolerance the patients have a normal existence.

The patient described by Coleman [1] required anaesthesia for caesarean section and refused a regional technique. Alcuronium was used to provide good intubating conditions—onset time was rapid and good recovery achieved. Suxamethonium was avoided because of the risk of myoglobinuria. Vecuronium or atracurium were suggested as better agents but were not available (Rajah and Bell [2] used atracurium without adverse effect). To provide substrate for muscle metabolism dextrose was given intraoperatively and continued for 24 hours afterwards—no muscle fatigue was experienced.

Tourniquets should be avoided as ischaemia may produce muscular atrophy; the patients should not be allowed to become cold as they have a limited ability to generate heat by shivering and in the elderly the reduced muscular power could lead to respiratory insufficiency.

References

1 Coleman P. *Anaesthesia,* 1984; **39:** 784−787.
2 Rajah A, Bell CF. *Anaesthesia,* 1986; **41:** 93.

Further reading

Cox JM. *Anesthesiology,* 1968; **29:** 1221−1225.

Glycogen storage disease IX

Major problems
Hypoglycaemia on fasting
Ketoacidosis

The patient described [1] was thought to have type IX of the glycogen storage disease on clinical grounds. Type IX is the result of a deficiency of hepatic phosphorylase kinase—an enzyme that converts inactive phosphorylase b to phosophorylase a which then converts glycogen to glucose-1-phosphate. There are two variants: IXa is inherited in an autosomal recessive manner and IXb is a sex-linked recessive. Hepatomegaly, growth retardation and hypoglycaemia when fasting are the main features.

During the anaesthetic the patient became hypermetabolic and developed a pyrexia and a metabolic acidosis. It is suggested that similar patients undergoing anaesthesia should have both lactic acid and ketoacids measured.

Reference

1 Edelstein G, Hirschman CA. *Anesthesiology,* 1980; **52:** 90−92.

Haemolytic uraemic syndrome

Major problems
Anaemia
Renal failure
Coagulopathy

This syndrome of renal failure, haemolytic anaemia and thrombocytopaenia, is found most often in children between the age of one and two years. A viral infection is thought to be the triggering event. It is a multisystem disease involving all the major organs. Haemorrhagic gastritis, myocarditis, liver dysfunction, coma and pulmonary insufficiency are all possible. Renal function may, or may not, return to normal.

It is important that the patient has a thorough medical assessment—the most important factors being anaemia, coagulopathy and renal failure. An attempt should be made to correct deficits where possible and anaesthesia should be undertaken using minimally disruptive agents and techniques. Care should be taken with the choice of muscle relaxants—with both liver and renal dysfunction atracurium may be the drug of choice. Monitoring should be intensive and include regular measurements of acid-base and electrolyte status. The commonest procedure performed is the formation of an arterio-venous shunt for dialysis.

Reference

1 Johnson GD, Rosales JK. *Can. J. Anaesth.*, 1987; **34:** 196−199.

Haemophilia A and B

Christmas disease

Major problem
Bleeding

A deficiency of factor VIII results in haemophilia A; it is a sex-linked recessive condition. Although the female carrier commonly has normal coagulation, Inwood and Meltzer [1] described three patients with clinically important bleeding tendencies. A deficiency of factor IX (Christmas factor) results in haemophilia B.

Management of these patients is primarily the management of the coagulopathy. Factor VIII or IX concentrate should be given in adequate amounts to ensure normal coagulation. The first dose should be given 2 hours prior to surgery, another infusion following surgery and additional doses 8 hourly for up to five days. Further doses are recommended 12 hourly until the patient is discharged from hospital.

Sampson et al. [2] reported the safety of local anaesthetic blocks (two axillary blocks) and the absence of complications following tracheal intubation.

Cryoprecipitate contains fibrinogen and this fibrinogen may increase the bleeding in the presence of adequate levels of factor VIII. It is recommended that the commercially available concentrate is used. These are usually supplied under the direct supervision of a haematologist and it is wise to involve the haematologists at an early stage.

References

1 Inwood MJ, Meltzer DB. *Can. Anaesth. Soc. J.*, 1978; **25**: 266–269.
2 Sampson JF, Hamstra R, Aldrete JA. *Anesth. Analg.*, 1979; **58**: 133–135.

Hallerman-Streiff syndrome

Oculomandibulodyscephaly with hypotrichosis

Major problems
Airway difficulty
Mental retardation

The Hallerman-Streiff syndrome is a result of maldevelopment at about the 5th or 6th week of embryonic life. Some chromosomal abnormalities have been described. Of significance to the anaesthetist is the hypoplastic nose with septal deviation, microstomia, high arched palate and mandibular hypoplasia. The temporomandibular joint is usually abnormal and together with the abnormally shaped brittle teeth, tracheal intubation can be exceedingly difficult. Proportionate dwarfism, scoliosis, osteoporosis and hyperextensible joints also cause problems and mental retardation reduces patient cooperation.

The patient described [1] was to undergo caesarean section. Tracheal intubation was carried out with the patient awake following the administration of an antacid. Both the oral and nasal routes were prepared using topical local anaesthetic solution and a 5.5 mm tracheal tube was used with a stylet. Anaesthesia was otherwise uneventful.

Regional anaesthesia was avoided because of her scoliosis, short stature making height of block unpredictable, and her impaired ability to cooperate.

Reference

1 Ravindran R, Stoops CM. *Anesth. Analg.*, 1979; **58**: 254—255.

Heart block

Stokes-Adams attacks

Major problem
Sudden cardiac arrest

First degree heart block is defined as a prolongation of the PR interval beyond 0.2 seconds. Second degree heart block is present when not every atrial beat is conducted through to the ventricles. Third degree (complete) heart block is characterised by complete atrioventricular dissociation. The latter results in a ventricular rate of about 40 beats per minute and often causes subjective symptoms of dizziness and syncope (Stokes-Adams attacks).

The importance of heart block to anaesthesia is that most anaesthetic agents possess some depressant action upon the myocardium and the myocardial conduction system. First and second degree blocks are thus very likely to change to third degree blocks and third degree blocks to asystole. It is therefore essential that the patients have a temporary pacing wire inserted pre-operatively if they do not already have a permanent implanted demand pacemaker. In cases where unexpected complete heart block develops intra-operatively, full cardiac resuscitative measures are clearly immediately indicated. Isoprenaline by infusion should maintain the cardiac output until a temporary pacing wire can be inserted. Pulmonary flotation catheters with inbuilt pacing electrodes are also available and an external cardiac pacing device has recently been introduced. A high index of suspicion should be maintained for all patients with otherwise unexplained episodes of fainting or dizziness.

Further reading

Ross EDT. *Br. J. Anaesth.*, 1962; **34:** 102–106.

Heerfordts syndrome
Uveoparotid fever

Major problem
Facial paralysis

Heerfordts syndrome is a form of sarcoidosis presenting with uveitis, parotitis, mild fever and cranial nerve palsies. The facial nerve is affected in 50−70% of patients. Steroids should be used early to prevent permanent nerve damage.

The patient described [1] developed a facial paralysis following a 'mask anaesthetic'. The weakness of the face was initially thought to be due to mechanical pressure during the procedure but the diagnosis was eventually made when the uveitis developed.

Reference

1 Vaghadia H. *Anesthesiology*, 1986; **64:** 513−514.

Hereditary angioedema

Major problem
Airway obstruction

Hereditary angioedema is an autosomal dominant disorder where oedema formation occurs spontaneously or as a result of trauma or emotional stress. The primary defect is a deficiency of the inhibitor of the first component of the complement cascade. Formation of oedema can occur quickly and at any site; about a quarter of the deaths in this disease are associated with respiratory obstruction. This is *not* an allergic condition and does *not* respond to antihistamines or adrenaline. The acute management of this oedema is the infusion of fresh frozen plasma which has adequate amounts of C_1 inhibitor to terminate an attack. There is the theoretical problem of supplying further substrates for the production of kinins that may increase capillary permeability but this does not seem to be a practical problem.

Anaesthesia in this condition is potentially hazardous—prophylactic fresh frozen plasma should be given and all procedures carried out with the absolute minimum amount of trauma. Long-term prophylaxis is with either epsilon aminocaproic acid or tranexamic acid, both of which have a C_1 inhibitor sparing effect. They do, however, carry the risk of intravascular thrombosis. They are also of value in the acute attacks.

Further reading

Hamilton AG, Bosley ARJ, Bowen DJ. *Anaesthesia*, 1977; **32**: 265−267.
Hopkinson RB, Sutcliffe AJ. *Anaesthesia*, 1979; **34**: 183−186.

Heredopathia atactica polyneuritiformis

Refsum's disease

Major problem
Peripheral neuropathy

This is an extremely rare autosomal recessive disorder involving the metabolism of a fatty acid—phytanic acid. Phytanic acid is normally converted to alpha-hydroxyphytanic acid but the enzyme alpha-hydroxylase is deficient. Phytanic acid accumulates in tissue lipids and produces symptoms of a progressive sensori-motor peripheral neuropathy, retinitis pigmentosa and ichthyosis.

The patient reported by Cullen [1] was anaesthetised using thiopentone followed by nitrous oxide and halothane in oxygen— without any adverse effect. No other reported cases have been found in the anaesthetic literature. Precautions as with other peripheral neuropathies are advised. Cullen stresses possible respiratory paralysis and cardiac conduction defects.

Reference

1 Cullen SC. *Anesthesiology*, 1962; **23**: 269−271.

Hippopotamus face

Fibro-osseous dysplasia of jaws

Major problem
Airway control

This rare jaw 'tumour', a developmental abnormality not a neo-plasm, arises from the alveolar margins of the upper and lower jaws and is so proliferative that it protrudes from the mouth, severely distorting the lips and eventually occluding the nostrils. Feeding and drinking are difficult.

The reference describes two brothers who had the condition [1]. Their father also had the condition and his tumour was excised twenty years previously, following the performance of a tracheostomy. Each child was intubated (one by blind nasal intubation and the other with the aid of an intubating rigid bronchoscope) and the surgery was carried out in four stages at 2−3 weekly intervals.

Reference

1 Kundu JP, Pan AK. *Br. J. Anaesth.*, 1979; **51**: 465−467.

Homocystinuria

Major problem
Thromboembolism

Homocystinuria results from a deficiency of cystathionine synthetase—this enzyme is involved in the transulphuration of the precursors of cysteine and its deficiency leads to a weakening of collagen. It is inherited in an autosomal recessive manner and its general incidence is 1:200 000—in Ireland, however, it is five times more common. Clinically the patient suffers the effects of lens dislocation, lax ligaments, kyphoscoliosis and other orthopaedic dysfunctions due to the weakened collagen. Mental retardation results if diagnosis and therapy are delayed—homocystine levels can be reduced by a low methionine content diet and the administration of pyridoxine, which is a co-enzyme in the metabolic pathway of methionine.

The major problem associated with surgery is the tendency to thromboembolism. The aetiology of this is debated but one hypothesis is that fraying collagen in vessel walls leads to loss of endothelial cells and this induces intravascular clotting; another is that homocystine may activate the Hageman (contact) factor.

All three case reports stress the importance of decreasing platelet adhesiveness, pyridoxine therapy and dextran 70, avoiding dehydration, maintaining the cardiac output at a high level and systemic vascular resistance at a low level, ensuring good venous flow (calf massage or stockings) and early ambulation.

Local anaesthetic blocks near major vessels, or in the spinal canal, should be considered carefully as damaged vessels or paralysed limbs with stagnant circulation may result in catastrophic thrombosis.

Further reading

Crooke JW, Towers JF, Taylor WH. Br. J. Anaesth., 1971; **43**: 96−99.
Grover VK, Malhotra SK, Kaushik S. Anaesthesia, 1979; **34**: 913−914.
Parris WCV, Quimby CW. Anesth. Analg., 1982; **61**: 708−710.

Huntington's chorea

Major problems
Possible sensitivity to thiopentone
Possible abnormal pseudocholinesterase

The incidence of this inherited autosomal dominant disease is about 7:100 000. It makes itself apparent at about 35–40 years of age and progresses relentlessly until death. Degeneration of the nerve cells of the basal ganglion and cerebral cortex results in forgetfulness and restlessness (early symptoms), involuntary movements of face, head and hands, ataxia, slurred speech and finally dementia.

There has been much debate in the literature about the apparent prolonged effect of thiopentone in patients with Huntington's chorea [1, 2]. The prolonged apnoea could well have been due to the very large dose of thiopentone given or to the presence of the rare fluoride resistant gene which has now been shown to be more common in these patients.

The patient may be on a wide range of drugs and care should be exercised to avoid interactions. Haloperidol, diazepam, reserpine, lithium, L-dopa, and chlordiazepoxide are a common selection.

Many anaesthetic agents have been used without problems, including suxamethonium, and as long as the appropriate dose for the debilitated patient is used problems are unlikely.

References

1 Blanloeil Y, Bigot A, Dixneuf B. *Anaesthesia,* 1982; **37**: 695–696.
2 Davies DD. *Br. J. Anaesth.,* 1966; **38**: 490–491.

Further reading

Browne MG. *Anaesthesia,* 1983; **38**: 65–66.
Farina J, Rauscher LA. *Br. J. Anaesth.,* 1977; **49**: 1167–1168.
Lamont AMS. *Anaesth. Intensive Care,* 1979; **7**: 189–190.
Lamont AMS. *Anaesth. Intensive Care,* 1981; **9**: 179.
Lamont ASM. *Anaesthesia,* 1983; **38**: 295.
Wells D. *Anaesth. Intensive Care,* 1979; **7**: 383–384.

Hyperaldosteronism

Conn's syndrome

Major problems
Hypokalaemia
Hypertension

Hyperaldosteronism may be primary (Conn's syndrome), due to an adenoma in the adult or hyperplasia in the juvenile, or it may be secondary to malignant or reno-vascular hypertension. The two problems of great concern to the anaesthetist are the severe hypokalaemia and hypertension. Spironolactone, an aldosterone antagonist, is the mainstay of pre-operative preparation together with potassium supplementation. Most of the clinical problems arise from potassium dysequilibrium; total potassium replacement is said to be virtually impossible.

Levy's patient [1], undergoing caesarean section, was given an infusion of potassium and the baby was delivered in a flaccid state (K^+ 7.3 mmol l^{-1})—the placenta provides no barrier to the potassium. Gangat's patient [2] was given potassium and the abnormal transcellular potassium concentration gradient caused muscular hypertonicity on induction of anaesthesia. Anaesthesia was terminated and following a more protracted potassium replacement regimen anaesthesia was successfully accomplished.

Shipton and Hugo [3] recommend an infusion of 6 mmol h^{-1} of potassium for 24 hours pre-operatively and intra-operatively. Their patient required another 20 g of potassium chloride in the first 12 hours following surgery.

Finch [4] reported on 60 patients, over half of which had systolic pressures in excess of 200 mmHg and a third had systolic pressures over 225 mmHg. A quarter of the patients had a hypertensive response to tumour manipulation but only two required intervention—one with phentolamine and the other with chlorpromazine.

Suxamethonium was used by most authors, even in the presence of potassium dysequilibrium, without adverse effect. Glucose intolerance is found in over half the patients with hyperaldosteronism and a search should therefore be made for this problem pre-operatively. Replacement steroid therapy is only required if both adrenals are removed. Patients in an uncontrolled state may be hypovolaemic and have a hypokalaemic alkalosis with muscle weakness, tetany and paraesthesia.

References

1 Levy J, Marx GF. *Anesthesiology*, 1971; **34:** 294−297.
2 Gangat Y, Triner L, Baer L, Puchner P. *Anesthesiology*, 1976; **45:** 542−544.
3 Shipton EA, Hugo JM. *Anaesthesia*, 1982; **37:** 933−936.
4 Finch JS. *Br. J. Anaesth.*, 1969; **41:** 880−883.

Hypercalcaemia

Hyperparathyroidism, pseudohyperparathyroidism

Major problems
Elevated serum calcium
Altered response to neuromuscular blocking
  agents

Hypercalcaemia may result from a number of causes including hyperparathyroidism and pseudohyperparathyroidism. Hyperparathyroidism is the result of an adenoma in most cases, or due to gland hypertrophy. Pseudohyperparathyroidism follows the production of a type of parathyroid stimulating hormone in association with certain malignancies. The patients are usually dehydrated, with impaired renal function. They are at risk from sudden cardiac arrest. Treatment with sodium-containing intravenous fluids and frusemide is appropriate. Thiazide diuretics should be avoided.

Serum calcium concentration should be brought down, preferably to within normal limits, before anaesthesia. Tolerance to any given calcium level varies widely from patient to patient and it is the ionised fraction which is important. It is therefore not possible to give an absolute upper limit for safe anaesthesia. A neurolept technique has been used successfully and it has been suggested that volatile agents are best avoided. The use of muscle relaxants in the presence of an abnormal calcium level is safe but their duration of action may be unpredictable. One report [1] describes a patient who received both suxamethonium and atracurium. The former lasted a long time (16 minutes, although the plasma cholinesterase level was found to be low) and the latter lasted a shorter time than expected. The end tidal CO_2 should be monitored continuously and normocapnia maintained because changes in acid-base balance may alter the ionised/non-ionised calcium ratio.

Reference

1 Al-Mohaya S, Naguib M, Abdelatif M, Farag H. *Anesthesiology,* 1986; **65:** 554−557.

Further reading

Sealey MM. *Anaesthesia,* 1985; **40:** 170−177.

Hypercholinesterasaemia

Major problem
Poor response to suxamethonium

Hypercholinesterasaemia can occur as a result of obesity, diabetes mellitus, hyperthyroidism or the nephrotic syndrome. It can also occur during the recovery from hepatitis. Hypercholinesterasaemia can be inherited, a condition which is thought to be transmitted in a dominant manner.

The patient described [1] responded poorly, on two occasions, to suxamethonium and was found to have serum cholinesterase concentrations more than twice normal.

Reference

1 Warran P, Theeman M, Bold AM, Jones S. *Anaesthesia*, 1987; **42**: 855–857.

Hypereosinophilic syndrome

Major problems
Cardiac failure
Hypercoagulation

The hypereosinophilic syndrome is the end product of any disease process that causes an excessive release of eosinophils into the circulation. Major organs may be infiltrated by the cells. Cardiac involvement occurs in over half of the patients and mural thrombosis sometimes causes systemic embolisation.

The patient described [1] was undergoing mitral and tricuspid valve replacement and required large doses of heparin to maintain blood fluidity. The activated clotting time was used to monitor anticoagulation because it seemed to correlate the best with the absence of clot. It is recommended that the activated clotting time should be greater than 300 seconds.

Reference

1 Hanowell ST, Kim YD, Rattan V, MacNamara TE. *Anesthesiology*, 1981; **55**: 450−452.

Hyperinsulinism

Major problem

Hypoglycaemia

This condition is the result of a benign or malignant tumour of the beta cells of the islets of Langerhans in the pancreas. The symptomatology is that of hypoglycaemia with excessive autonomic activity, changes in behaviour and convulsions.

Dangerous hypoglycaemia can be avoided by the regular administration of oral glucose (50 g two hourly) in the pre-operative period and by the infusion of strong dextrose solutions intra-operatively through a central venous catheter. Handling of the tumour may cause acute falls in blood sugar and thus the blood sugar level should be monitored very closely. The EEG can alternatively be used to detect the cerebral effects of hypoglycaemia although this technique requires familiarity with such EEG changes.

Postoperative hyperglycaemia is usual and it may take several days for the blood sugar to fall. Insulin is not usually required.

Further reading

Bourke AM. *Anaesthesia*, 1966; **21**: 239−243.
Chari P, Pandit SK, Kataria RN, Singh DK, Wig J. *Anaesthesia*, 1977: **32**: 261−264.
Fraser RA. *Anaesthesia*, 1963; **18**: 3−8.
Hargadon JJ, Ormston TOG. *Br. J. Anaesth.*, 1963; **35**: 807−810.

Hyperlipoproteinaemia

Major problem
Thrombosis

Hyperlipoproteinaemia increases the risk of platelet aggregation and thrombosis. The patient described [1] developed acute pancreatitis and was in circulatory failure; a combination of indwelling radial arterial cannula, a dopamine infusion, hyperlipoproteinaemia, hyperosmolarity (glucose 700 mg dl^{-1} or 38 mmol l^{-1}), hypovolaemia and capillary sludging led to gangrene of the cannulated forearm necessitating amputation.

If the risk of thrombosis is high, avoid cannulating small arteries.

Reference

1 Cannon BW, Meshier WT. *Anesthesiology*, 1982; **56**: 222−223.

Hypermagnesaemia

Major problems
Muscular weakness
Coma

Hypermagnesaemia is usually iatrogenic. The management of eclampsia with magnesium sulphate and then the subsequent anaesthesia for caesarean section are the scenarios for the two case reports referenced [1, 2]. Hypermagnesaemia may occur in advanced renal disease. The normal plasma magnesium concentration is between 0.75 and 1.25 mmol 1^{-1}. That in Skaredoff's patient [2] was 4.0 mmol 1^{-1} and that in De Silva's patient [1] was 3.5 mmol 1^{-1}.

One patient had suxamethonium and spontaneous respiration occurred three hours later (plasma cholinesterase was within normal limits) and the other patient had suxamethonium followed by tubocurarine on return of respiratory activity. This patient was extubated after one hour but showed signs of incomplete reversal of muscular paralysis; she was observed closely and at three hours could lift her limbs and head normally. Magnesium also affects cardiac rhythmicity and uterine muscle — high levels are associated with diminished contractions. High levels may also produce a comatose state.

References

1 De Silva AJC. *Br. J. Anaesth.*, 1973; **45:** 1228–1229.
2 Skaredoff MN, Roaf ER Datta S. *Can. Anaesth. Soc. J.*, 1982; **29:** 35–41.

Further reading

Paymaster NJ. *Ann. R. Coll. Surg. (Eng.)*, 1976; **58:** 309–314.

Hyperreninism

Major problems
Hypertension
Hypokalaemia

Hyperreninism is the result of either renal ischaemia or neoplasia of the juxtaglomerular apparatus and presents as hypertension, hypokalaemia and hyperaldosteronism. The diagnosis depends on the finding of raised renin levels in the renal vein. Nephrectomy is the treatment.

The report referenced [1] stresses the management of the hypertension (sodium nitroprusside was used) but does not mention the hypokalaemia. Hypertensive crises can be precipitated by the manipulation of the kidney. Release of extra angiotension II, as a result of the high renin levels, stimulates the release of catecholamines from the adrenal medulla and thus agents that sensitise the myocardium to catecholamines should be avoided.

Reference

1 Christian CM, Naraghi M. *Anesthesiology,* 1977; **46:** 436−437.

Hyperthyroidism (uncontrolled)

Major problems
Hyperdynamic cardiovascular system
Hypermetabolic state

Patients undergoing thyroid surgery are usually euthyroid but there are a small minority who either require urgent coincidental surgery or cannot take the medication required to make them euthyroid. This small minority can present a grave risk. It must be emphasised that, if possible, hyperthyroidism should be investigated and controlled to render the patient euthyroid before anaesthesia is considered.

Adrenergic blocking agents are used to control the symptoms and signs and iodine may be used to produce a temporary reduction in thyroid hormone formation and a decrease in the gland's vascularity. The patient should be well sedated prior to surgery (a benzodiazepine is satisfactory) and anaesthesia should be induced with thiopentone (it is known to have an antithyroid action). Maintenance of anaesthesia with a neurolept anaesthetic regimen would seem least likely to upset the thryoid/adrenal axis and avoiding the volatile inhalational agents may avoid the complexity of catecholamine related dysrhythmias.

Thyroid 'storm' occurs 6−18 hours postoperatively and thus the patient should be closely monitored. Aggressive management with anti-thyroid drugs, steroids and adrenergic blocking agents is required. It may be initiated by infection, palpation of the goitre or acute iodine withdrawal.

Further reading

Stehling LC. *Anesthesiology*, 1974; **41**: 585−595.
Kadis LB, Bennett EJ, Dalal FY, Zander HL. *Anesth. Analg.*, 1966; **45**: 415−421.

119

Hypophosphataemia

Major problems
Muscle weakness
Coma

Plasma phosphate concentration is determined by renal re-absorption. It is low in renal tubular disorders and may also be affected by drugs—particularly corticosteroids. Intravenous saline causes increased phosphate excretion.

Severe hypophosphataemia is treated by the infusion of di-potassium hydrogen phosphate; the recommended dose is 0.08 mmol kg^{-1} every 6 hours but this dose may need to be exceeded to maintain body stores. The complications of high dose infusion include hypocalcaemia, hypotension, hyperkalaemia, hyper-natraemia and dehydration.

Further reading

Lindsay SL, Mason DF. *Anaesthesia,* 1987; **42:** 439.

Hypothyroidism

Myxoedema, cretinism

Major problems
Sensitivity to anaesthetic agents
Hypothermia

Hypothyroidism may exist without the overt signs of myxoedema—coarse, sparse hair, dry skin, oedema, cardiac failure and coma. The disease is one of great variability. A low thyroxine level and an elevated cholesterol are adequate for the initial diagnosis. Patients should be made euthyroid before elective surgery; this will take two weeks.

Hypotension, hypothermia and slow recovery are the three common findings in hypothyroid patients undergoing anaesthesia. The use of inhalational agents rather than intravenous ones has been recommended [1] although the development of newer intravenous agents may modify this advice.

Reference

1 Kim JM, Hackman L. *Anesth. Analg.*, 1977; **56**: 299–302.

Idiopathic pulmonary haemosiderosis

Major problems
Anaemia
Hypoxia

Recurrent haemorrhage into the lung is the main overt sign of idiopathic pulmonary haemosiderosis. The patient is usually hypoxaemic due to pulmonary consolidation and may be severely anaemic; the disease is very variable in its severity. These patients usually present for anaesthesia for a diagnostic open lung biopsy. They may be very sick and time should be spent improving their general condition—primarily transfusion and oxygen therapy. In the acute phase corticosteroids are helpful.

It is thought that the cause of the disease may be a disruption of the basement membrane associated with the type 2 pneumatocytes. Airway pressures should be kept to a minimum as high airway pressures are thought to exacerbate the derangement of the basement membrane. High frequency jet ventilation may be preferable to conventional ventilation if ventilatory support is necessary.

With the haemorrhagic tendency (in the presence of normal clotting) the endotracheal tube can become occluded with clot and should be regularly checked. Humidification and regular bronchial toilet is advised. A myocarditis has been reported with the condition and thus cardiac performance should be closely monitored.

Further reading

Whitehurst P, Page RL, Will EJ. *Anaesthesia*, 1985; **40**: 37−41.

Infantile lobar emphysema

Major problems
Hypoxaemia
Hypotension

The lobar emphysema in the patients described caused contralateral pulmonary compression due to the mediastinal shift. This is the typical presentation which is associated with infection, dyspnoea and tachypnoea. The cardiovascular system may be compromised by the mediastinal shift but there may also be a congenital abnormality of the heart (10%).

Surgical excision of the lobe is the treatment of choice and may be required urgently. It has been suggested by Cote [1] that anaesthesia should be maintained with the patient breathing spontaneously so as to minimise airway pressures thus exacerbating an already difficult situation. Should the emphysematous lung become acutely distended the thorax should be opened quickly to allow the intrathoracic pressure to fall and venous return to improve. Volatile agents appeared to aggravate the cardiovascular decompensation and are probably best avoided, as is nitrous oxide which may also increase the size of the emphysematous lobe.

Ketamine, with local anaesthetic infiltration, is advocated as a possible technique until the chest is opened. Kwik's patient [2] required prolonged respiratory support following the lobectomy. Cote's patients were extubated at the end of surgery.

References

1 Cote CJ. *Anesthesiology*, 1974; **49**: 296−298.
2 Kwik RSH. *Br. J. Anaesth.*, 1977; **49**: 633−635.

Infectious mononucleosis

Major problem
Possible airway obstruction

In severe infectious mononucleosis the airway may be obstructed by swelling of any of the pharyngeal structures—from tonsils to arytenoids. They will be inflamed, infected, friable and likely to bleed easily.

The patient described [1] underwent emergency tonsillectomy and adenoidectomy for which a tracheal tube was passed orally under droperidol and atropine premedication and topical local anaesthetic. An alternative approach would have been an elective tracheostomy.

Reference

1 Meyers EF, Krupin B. *Anesthesiology*, 1975; **42**: 490−491.

Jaw winking syndrome

Marcus Gunn syndrome

Major problem
Dysrhythmia

An abnormal connection between the trigeminal and the oculo-motor nerves causes the eyelid to retract when the jaw is moved.

The normal oculocardiac reflex occurs in response to pressure on the eyeball, to traction on the extra-ocular muscles and to raised intra-ocular pressure. Sinus bradycardia, junctional rhythms, atrio-ventricular block and asystole are all possible. Kwik's patient [1] developed dysrhythmias on handling of the eyelid and the dysrhythmias were premature atrial contractions with a wandering pacemaker. He postulated that patients with the Marcus Gunn syndrome were "more prone to develop an atypical oculocardiac reflex due to the existence of abnormal central connexions".

He advised that all such patients should be closely monitored, that atropine be given at induction of anaesthesia and that controlled ventilation is preferable to spontaneous ventilation with a volatile agent.

Reference

1 Kwik RSH. *Anaesthesia*, 1980; **35**: 46−49.

Juvenile chronic polyarthritis

Still's disease

Major problems
Potential airway obstruction
Limitation of neck movement

In this condition there is marked limitation of extension of the neck and sometimes the vertebral bodies may be fused. The possibility of atlanto-axial subluxation should be considered. Other skeletal abnormalities may limit positioning of the patient or further impede airway management—the lower jaw may recede and produce an abnormal bite which together with restriction of the jaw movement may make conventional orotracheal intubation impossible.

D'Arcy *et al.* [1] make a strong recommendation for the use of ketamine and nitrous oxide in oxygen for major orthopaedic surgery. They advise that cricothyroid puncture may still be necessary to maintain oxygenation in the worst patients as airway obstruction can still occur.

Dennison [2] and Smith [3] described fibre-optic laryngoscopy and Hausdoerfer [4] blind nasal intubation with local anaesthesia. Greaves [5] advocates spinal or epidural anaesthesia.

The patient described by Campbell *et al.* [6] was a 14-year-old with juvenile rheumatoid arthritis who suffered hepatic necrosis following a halothane anaesthetic.

References

1 D'Arcy EJ, Fell RH, Ansell BM, Arden GP. *Anaesthesia*, 1976; **31:** 624−632.
2 Dennison PH. *Br. J. Anaesth.*, 1978; **50:** 636.
3 Smith BL. *Anaesthesia*, 1985; **40:** 209.
4 Hausdoerfer J. *Br. J. Anaesth.*, 1979; **51:** 75.
5 Greaves JD. *Br. J. Anaesth.*, 1979; **51:** 75.
6 Campbell RL, Small EN, Lesesne HR, Levin KJ, Moore WH. *Anesth. Analg.*, 1977; **56:** 589−593.

Further reading

Hodgkinson R. *Anesth. Analg.*, 1981; **60:** 611−612.

126

Kawasaki disease

Mucocutaneous lymph node syndrome

Major problem
Cardiac dysfunction

The aetiology of this disease is unknown but it is most common in Japanese male children. It is thought to be the result of a systemic vasculitis that affects arteries and veins producing aneurysms, carditis, conduction disturbances and valvular lesions.

Coronary artery aneurysms are common and may require coronary artery surgery. Myocardial ischaemia is possible and the anaesthetic technique chosen should maintain the myocardial oxygen demand/supply ratio. It is advised that both leads II and V5 of the electrocardiogram are monitored. Cardiovascular stability is essential.

Aspirin and dipyridamole are used in combination to reduce aneurysm formation and prolong platelet function.

Further reading

McNiece WL, Krishna G. *Anesthesiology,* 1983; **58:** 269−271.

Klippel-Feil syndrome

Major problem
Cervical instability

Klippel-Feil's syndrome of a short neck (either fused cervical vertebrae or fewer verterbrae) and a low posterior hair line leads to limitation of neck movement with concomitant airway management problems. Other abnormalities are usually present and should be sought — skeletal, cardiovascular and genito-urinary anomalies are common.

Spinal cord injury at the cervical level is the greatest hazard during anaesthesia and positioning for surgery, and thus extreme care needs to be taken during airway maintenance and movement of the child.

The choice of anaesthetic agents is likely to be determined by the medical condition and a full assessment of all systems is therefore of utmost importance. About 10% of these patients have a cardiovascular anomaly.

Further reading

Naguib M, Farag H, Ibrahim AEW. *Can. Anaesth. Soc. J.*, 1986; **33**: 66—70.
Daum REO, Jones DJ. *Anaesthesia*, 1988; **43**: 18—21.

Larsen's syndrome

Major problem
Possible difficult intubation

Larsen's syndrome is characterised by multiple congenital joint dislocations, usually bilateral, affecting elbows, hips, knees and shoulders. Patients have prominent foreheads with a flattened nasal bridge and wide-set eyes. The basic congenital defect is one of abnormal connective tissue formation leading to production of poor cartilage which lacks rigidity. This defective cartilage may also be found in the epiglottis, arytenoids, trachea and ribs. Patients with Larsen's syndrome are likely to have other congenital disorders, in particular congenital heart lesions and cleft palate.

The patients may present problems with tracheal intubation and appropriate precautions must therefore be taken. Chronic respiratory symptoms are also a common feature and the patient may suffer an acute exacerbation during the postoperative period. Positioning the patient must be performed with care due to the laxity of many of the major joints.

Further reading

Larsen LJ, Schottstaedt ER, Bost FC. *J. Ped.*, 1950: **37**: 574–581.
Robertson FW, Kozlowski K, Middleton RW. *Clin. Pediat.*, 1975; **14**: 53–60.

Laryngeal papillomatosis

Major problems

Avoid trauma to lesions on intubation

Beware postoperative laryngeal oedema

Small benign papillomatous growths appear on the true vocal cords and need regular surgical removal. They appear at age 12 to 18 months and commonly regress spontaneously around puberty. Although usually confined to the vocal cords the growths may spread to the trachea and bronchi (tracheobronchial papillomatosis). The patients usually present with hoarseness, dyspnoea or stridor. Chronic partial airway obstruction may be present which may become acute if the lesions become infected. Pedunculated lesions within the lumen of the trachea or bronchi may obstruct the entrance to smaller bronchi.

The safest technique of anaesthesia is inhalational induction with maintenance of anaesthesia spontaneously breathing a volatile agent. Local analgesia spray may be applied to the larynx. A suspension laryngoscope, microscope and laser may be used by the surgeon, in which case precautions appropriate to laser surgery apply. Laryngeal oedema may be a problem in the postoperative period [1]. This will be helped by a short course of steroids and humidification of inspired gases. It is best to avoid tracheal intubation or tracheostomy formation if possible because this may promote distal seeding of the papillomata [2].

References

1 Harper JR, Thomas K, Wirk H. *Anaesthesia*, 1973; **28:** 71−74.
2 Callander CC. *Anaesth. Intensive Care*, 1979; **51:** 201−202.

Laryngocoele

Major problems
Avoid positive pressure ventilation by mask
Intubate for all procedures

A laryngocoele is a pathological enlargement of a laryngeal ventricle where a closed sac forms adjacent to the larynx and which communicates with the larynx. These may appear at any age, classically occurring in players of wind instruments. The sac dilates when inflated with air, resulting in a swelling appearing in the neck. They are usually asymptomatic, although the size may be sufficient to cause intermittent symptoms of hoarseness, dyspnoea and dysphagia. If the laryngocoele contains a collection of fluid (which may become infected) this may subsequently spill out and soil the airway. It should be possible to estimate the size and position of a laryngocoele by anteroposterior and lateral soft tissue X-rays of the neck.

Positive pressure ventilation using a face-mask should be avoided because the laryngocoele will become inflated making subsequent laryngoscopy and intubation more difficult. An inhalational induction is therefore recommended. It may also be wise to undertake this with the patient in the lateral position, head down, so that any fluid displaced from the sac does not enter the patient's airway. The entrance to the sac is above the cricoid ring and so the application of cricoid pressure is unlikely to prevent fluid or air entering or leaving the sac. Care must be taken at intubation to ensure that the tracheal tube passes down the trachea and does not enter the sac.

Further reading

Divekar VM, Kavadia IP, Jhalla S. *Can. Anaesth. Soc. J.*, 1979, **26;** 140–141.

Laryngotracheo-oesophageal cleft

Major problems
Avoid positive pressure ventilation with mask
Possibility of tracheal tube entering cleft

This is a rare congenital anomaly characterised by absence of fusion of the posterior laminae of the cricoid cartilage. The result is an abnormal communication between the larynx and the hypopharynx or oesophagus. This communication may not be confined solely to the larynx but may extend for any distance from larynx to carina. A mild form has been described where absence of the interarytenoid muscle was the only abnormality, the patient suffering a hoarse voice and recurrent chest infections. It usually presents in the neonatal period with respiratory and feeding difficulties and requires urgent repair. Twenty per cent of the patients have additional major congenital abnormalities.

Repair of the defect usually requires surgery through the patient's airway with the aid of a microscope and suspension laryngoscope. If the cleft is extensive, a preliminary tracheostomy under local anaesthesia and a thoracotomy may be necessary. In addition to the usual precautions appropriate to the neonate, a technique using spontaneous respiration with a volatile agent is recommended. Premedication with atropine to dry secretions and spraying the larynx with lignocaine will also help. Positive pressure ventilation with a face-mask should be avoided because if there is free communication with the oesophagus the stomach will become distended further embarrassing respiration. Pre-operative intubation is likely to be difficult because the tracheal tube can pass through the defect into the oesophagus. If pre-operative intubation is required it may be necessary to first introduce a guidewire into the trachea using a bronchoscope and then to pass the tracheal tube over this guidewire.

Postoperatively a nasotracheal tube should be inserted and left *in situ* for several days until operative oedema has subsided.

Further reading

Armitage EN. *Anaesthesia*, 1984; **39:** 706−713.

Kingston HGG, Harrison MW, Smith JD. *Anesth. Analg.*, 1983; **62:** 1041−1043.

Ruder CB, Glaser LC. *Anesthesiology*, 1977; **47:** 65−66.

Yamashita M, Chinyanga HM, Steward DJ. *Can. Anaesth. Soc. J.*, 1979; **26:** 502−505.

Leigh's syndrome

Subacute necrotising encephalomyelopathy

Major problems
None

Leigh's syndrome is a chronic neurological disease presenting in infancy. Features include weakness, ataxia, convulsions and external ophthalmoplegia together with difficulties in feeding, swallowing and breathing. It follows a chronic relapsing course though acute exacerbations may occur following surgery. The metabolic defect is probably a deficiency in activation of pyruvate dehydrogenase enzyme leading to elevation in blood lactate and pyruvate concentrations.

No particular anaesthetic agent or technique is contraindicated. Close attention should be paid to airway management and temperature regulation because brainstem lesions may be present, affecting their central control. Excessive hyperventilation should be avoided because a reduction in pH has been reported to increase lactate production. It may be wise to avoid lactate containing intravenous fluids (e.g. Hartmann's solution).

Further reading

Ward DS. *Anesthesiology,* 1981; **55**: 80−81.

Lesch-Nyhan syndrome

Major problems
Renal insufficiency
Increased risk of tracheal aspiration
Increased sensitivity to catecholamines

In the Lesch-Nyhan syndrome there is a hereditary enzyme defect which results in abnormal purine metabolism. There is excess purine production and a raised level of uric acid. It is inherited in a sex-linked recessive manner and therefore only affects males. Patients are mentally subnormal and often suffer from spasticity of the limbs. Urinary calculi develop with nephropathy and subsequent renal failure. Seizure disorders and arthritis are also common.

In view of the likelihood of renal insufficiency a pre-operative assessment of renal function is necessary. If renal function is impaired, then drugs which are eliminated by that route should be avoided or administered with care. There is often a tendency to self-mutilation activity in these patients. When this has affected the mouth, gums, and face, difficulties may arise with the airway and intubation. It is unlikely that any anaesthetic agents rely on the defective enzyme pathway for their metabolism. The following agents have been said to present no problem [1]: thiopentone, methohexitone, etomidate, ketamine, isoflurane, atracurium, atropine and neostigmine. There is an increased risk of regurgitation of gastric contents and subsequent tracheal aspiration in these patients. Appropriate precautions must therefore be taken, particularly at induction and reversal. The arthritis and spasticity may make positioning of the patient difficult and this should be undertaken with great care.

The adrenergic pressor response to stress is blunted or absent. In addition there is a reduction in the level, or the activity, of monoamine oxidase. Exogenous catecholamines must be given very carefully and in reduced dosage, and it is wise to manage these patients as if they have monoamine oxidase inhibition.

Reference

1 Larson LO, Wilkins RG. *Anesthesiology*, 1985; **63**: 197–199.

Ludwig's angina

Major problems
Difficult airway management
Intubation problems

This is a potentially lethal, rapidly spreading cellulitis involving the floor of the mouth and spreading into the neck. The causative organism is usually a haemolytic streptococcus originating from an infected lower molar tooth or tonsil. Oedema of the pharynx is present with pain, dysphagia and trismus. The tongue is elevated and displaced posteriorly. Oedema of the larynx and vocal cords may also be present. Urgent treatment (antibiotics and surgical decompression) is important to prevent progression to mediastinitis and septicaemia.

The major problem faced by the anaesthetist is one of airway management. Serval options are available:

1 If swelling is extensive with severe trismus then the safest course of action is tracheostomy under local anaesthesia. However, this may be technically difficult due to tissue oedema in the neck. In addition, the effectiveness of local anaesthetic agents is impaired in inflamed tissues. Anaesthesia may then be induced by any appropriate means once the airway is secured.

2 Tracheal intubation may be performed with the patient awake using local anaesthesia. In view of the limited mouth opening, the nasal route will probably be necessary. If a fibreoptic laryngoscope is not available then a blind nasal intubation technique will have to be used. It is unwise to attempt this technique without previous experience. Once the airway is secured anaesthesia may be induced by any appropriate means.

3 Anaesthesia is induced using an inhalational technique. Spontaneous ventilation should be constantly maintained and muscle relaxants or narcotics avoided until tracheal intubation is secured. Once the patient is deeply anaesthetised sufficient relaxation may be present to allow the mouth to be opened enough for direct laryngoscopy to be performed. If this is still not possible, then the blind nasal or fibreoptic technique may have

to be attempted, or the patient awoken and a tracheostomy performed under local anaesthesia.

At all times when dealing with these patients full preparations for a difficult intubation should be made. A competent surgeon should also be continually standing by in order to perform an immediate tracheostomy should problems arise.

Further reading

Bevan DR, Monks PS, Calne DB. *Anaesthesia*, 1963; **28:** 29−31.
Loughnan TE, Allen DE. *Anaesthesia*, 1985; **40:** 295−297.

Lymphoma

Includes Burkitt's lymphoma; Hodgkin's disease

Major problems
Possible difficult intubation
Increased susceptibility to infection

Burkitt's lymphoma is a disease of children where rapidly growing lymphoid tumours appear. These are mainly situated around the mandibular and salivary glands although the adrenals, liver, heart and retro-peritoneal lymph nodes may also be affected.

Hodgkin's disease is principally a disorder affecting young adults although, like other non-Hodgkin's lymphomas, it may appear at any age. In these conditions there is a progressive, painless lymphadenopathy with nodes in the neck often the first to be involved. Other groups of nodes, mediastinal, axillary and abdominal, are also commonly affected. Secondary symptoms depend upon the site of these masses of enlarged nodes. Dysphagia, dyspnoea and venous obstruction have all been reported. The patients are often anaemic. Although the white cell count is elevated those cells do not function normally and the patient has an increased susceptibility to infections. They may also be receiving cytotoxic therapy which will further depress red cell count, white cell count and platelet numbers.

Lymphoid enlargements situated around the face and neck may lead to difficulties with intubation and appropriate precautions should be therefore be taken. Mediastinal lymph node enlargements may compress and distort the trachea, resulting in difficulty in advancing a tube down the trachea. Lymphoid enlargements in other sites are unlikely to affect anaesthesia. In view of the increased susceptibility to infection as much care as possible should be taken with venepuncture, intubation, etc. Reports have suggested that there may be an association between Burkitt's lymphoma and malignant hyperpyrexia. This link is tenuous, however, and of doubtful significance.

Further reading

Flewellen EH. *Anesth. Analg.,* 1980; **59:** 955.
Lees DE, Gadde PL, MacNamara TE. *Anesth. Analg.,* 1980; **59:** 514–515.
Tsueda K, Dubick MN, Wright BD, Sachatello CR. *Anesth. Analg.,* 1978; **57:** 511–514.

Lymphosarcoma cutis

Major problem
Frequent multiple general anaesthetics

Symptomless tumours appear on the skin in this condition which are histologically lymphosarcomas. The patient may also have leukaemia. It is a disease of children. Most patients die within six months and the five-year survival rate is only about 9−13%. The mainstays of treatment are cytotoxics and steroids.

Multiple general anaesthetics are needed for radiotherapy, biopsies and invasive diagnostic tests. In the case described [1], frequent general anaesthetics were performed using intramuscular ketamine and found to be very satisfactory. It is important to maintain sterility with all instrumentation in patients receiving cytotoxic therapy. Increased steroid doses in the perioperative period will be needed if on long-term steroid treatment.

Reference

1 Fynn RW. *Br. J. Anaesth.*, 1974; **46**: 699−700.

Malignant hyperpyrexia

Major problems
Hyperpyrexia and severe metabolic derangements
   triggered by a number of commonly used
   anaesthetic agents
Avoid triggering agents

Malignant hyperpyrexia (MH) is inherited in an autosomal dominant fashion with incomplete penetrance. If it is recognised in one member of a family it is important to screen all other close relatives of that person and to issue them with warning cards as appropriate. It has been recognised in patients ranging from age 6 months upwards but the commonest age of presentation is the second and third decades. Malignant hyperpyrexia appears to be a disorder of calcium flux within the muscle fibres such that there is a prolonged activation of the muscle contraction process. This can be triggered by a number of agents used in general anaesthesia and unless recognised and treated early will have serious or even fatal consequences. Associations have been reported with Duchenne muscular dystrophy, myotonica dystrophia, osteogenesis imperfecta, strabismus, kyphoscoliosis, congenital hernias, cleft palate and various other minor orthopaedic abnormalities. It is possible that the patient may have had a previous uneventful general anaesthetic, even involving one of the known trigger agents. Any family history of sudden deaths under anaesthesia should be viewed with the greatest suspicion. The mortality of this condition in patients not previously known to be at risk approaches 50%.

Once triggered, an MH reaction exhibits many but not all of the following features. Increased body temperature (may rise very rapidly—1°C every 15–20 minutes), skeletal muscle rigidity*, hyperventilation, hypercapnoea*, hypoxaemia (despite 100% oxygen therapy), cyanosis, tachycardia,* hypertension, cardiac arrythmias, hyperkalaemia, metabolic acidosis. Those marked with an asterisk are the most common early signs although the presentation is very unpredictable. Disseminated intravascular coagulation and renal failure may follow later.

Management of an MH crisis
Any volatile agent should be stopped and all vaporisers removed. The patient should be hyperventilated using 100% oxygen. Anaesthesia may be continued with one of the agents from the 'safe' list (see below) and the surgeon asked to complete the procedure as rapidly as possible. Continuous temperature monitoring should be started. Active cooling must be begun, including the infusion of cold intravenous fluids, irrigation of any readily available body cavity with cold fluids and packing ice around the patient especially in the axillae and groins. An arterial blood sample should be taken for blood gases and potassium. Dantrolene should be given in a dose of approximately 1 mg kg^{-1} IV, repeating as necessary up to a maximum total does of 10 mg kg^{-1}. Mannitol and fluids should be given to promote a diuresis. Dextrose should be given as part of the intravenous fluid regime. Arterial blood samples should be checked repeatedly and acidosis corrected with sodium bicarbonate and hyperkalaemia treated with glucose and insulin infusion. Dexamethasone (20 mg IV in an adult) has also been recommended, as has procaine (100 mg IV initially in an adult; maximum 30 mg kg^{-1}). Once the patient's body temperature has been returned to near normal and the metabolic derangements are under control the patient should be transferred to the intensive care unit for continued monitoring and treatment.

Subsequently it is most important that the patient be issued with a warning card and counselled appropriately. The patient should also be referred to the nearest MH investigation and advisory centre (Leeds in Great Britain) for further investigation and for the investigation of close relatives as appropriate.

Management of the known MH susceptible patient
Anaesthesia is safe provided that all known triggering agents are avoided and appropriate precautions taken in case of problems. In the pre-operative preparation of these patients dantrolene should be given orally for 24 hours in a dose of approximately 1 mg kg^{-1} every 6 hours. All vaporisers should be removed from

the anaesthetic machine, which should be well flushed through with oxygen. A new disposable anaesthetic circuit should be used. A supply of dantrolene for IV use should be available in the operating theatre before starting. An MH crisis may be triggered by many agents used in anaesthesia. The following should be **avoided:** volatile anaesthetic agents, suxamethonium and other depolarising agents, anticholinesterases, phenothiazines, ketamine, lignocaine, cyclopropane, atropine, tricyclic antidepressants, monoamine oxidase inhibitors. The following drugs are probably **safe:** nondepolarising muscle relaxants (pancuronium is recommended for use), fentanyl, droperidol, diazepam, procaine, thiopentone, nitrous oxide, bupivacaine, prilocaine.

There are many case reports in the literature, not all of which may be true MH. The reference list is not complete but is limited to a selection of the more recent reports and reviews.

Further reading

Ellis FR. *Br. J. Anaesth.*, 1980, **52;** 153−164.
Ellis FR, Halsall PJ, Harrison DGF. *Anaesthesia*, 1986, **41;** 809−815.
Fraser JG, Crumrine RS, Izant RJ. *Anesth. Analg.*, 1976, **55;** 713−718.
Gronert GA. *Anesthesiology*, 1980, **53;** 395−423.
Symposium on Malignant Hyperpyrexia. *Br. J. Anaesth.*, 1988, **60;** 251−319.

Mandibulofacial dysostosis

Treacher-Collins syndrome;
Pierre Robin syndrome

Major problems
Difficult airway maintenance
Difficult intubation

There are a number of rare syndromes covered by the term mandibulofacial dysostosis. Treacher-Collins syndrome is the most common. Pierre Robin syndrome does not strictly belong to this category but it is included due to similarity in management.

The Treacher-Collins syndrome results from a defect in the development of the first branchial arch. Resulting abnormalities include antimongoloid slanting eyes, absent eyelashes, coloboma of the eyelids, ear abnormalities (often with deafness), under-developed maxilla with high arched palate and a poorly developed mandible with receding chin. Additional minor skeletal abnormalities may occasionally be present.

The Pierre Robin syndrome consists of the combination of mandibular hypoplasia (micrognathia), macroglossia and cleft palate. Cardiovascular anomalies are relatively common in the Pierre Robin syndrome, septal defects or patent ductus arteriosus in particular. Eye, ear, or other abnormalities may additionally be present.

The most important problem with these patients is one of airway management and it is not uncommon for airway difficulties to be already present. A number of these patients may additionally suffer from sleep apnoeas. The simple act of placing the patient in the supine position may compromise the airway and it is often necessary to nurse these patients in the prone position to prevent the tongue from falling backwards. Airway and intubation difficulties should be expected in these patients. The facial deformity may be such that it is difficult to find a suitable face-mask. It may indeed be virtually impossible to maintain the airway in such patients, despite the aid of naso-pharyngeal or oropharyngeal airways. Respiratory depressant

144

drugs, intravenous anaesthetic agents and muscle relaxants are thus inadvisable until the airway is secure. Atropine premedication is useful but sedatives should be avoided or given with great care. It will therefore be necessary to intubate the patient awake, using topical local anaesthesia or under anaesthesia spontaneously breathing a volatile agent. The use of small doses of ketamine has also been shown to be a satisfactory technique. The following methods have all been used to secure tracheal intubation in these patients:

1 Blind nasal intubation.
2 Blind nasal intubation holding the patient prone with the neck hyperextended.
3 Blind oral intubation using a bougie.
4 Pulling out the tongue with forceps.
5 Fibroptic techniques (with or without the use of a guide wire).

Whichever technique is chosen it is wise to have a competent surgeon standing by to perform an urgent tracheostomy if required. It may even be appropriate to consider first performing an elective tracheostomy under local anaesthesia.

Postoperatively the patient should not be extubated until fully awake and the patient should be observed on a high dependency nursing unit for at least 24 hours. A tongue suture may be useful.

The airway problems must not divert attention from the rest of the patient. If there are co-existing cardiac lesions management appropriate to these must also be considered, including the use of prophylactic antibiotics.

Further reading

Divekar VM, Sircar BN. *Anesthesiology,* 1965; **26:** 692−693.
Howardy-Hansen P, Berthelsen P. *Anaesthesia,* 1988; **43:** 121.
MacLennan FM, Robertson GS. *Anaesthesia,* 1981; **36:** 196.
Miyabe M, Dohi S, Homma E. *Anesthesiology,* 1985, **62:** 213−215.
Rasch DK, Browder F, Barr M, Greer D. *Can. Anaesth. Soc. J.,* 1986, **33:** 364−370.
Roa NL, Moss KS. *Anesthesiology,* 1984, **60:** 71.
Sklar GS, King BD. *Anesthesiology,* 1976, **44:** 247.

Mastocytosis

Urticaria pigmentosa

Major problems
Hypotension and broncho-constriction from acute
massive histamine release

In this condition there are abnormal accumulations of mast cells throughout the body. These cells contain significant quantities of histamine, heparin and other vasoactive substances. Once release of these substances is triggered the patient suffers symptoms of urticaria, flushing, abdominal cramps, diarrhoea, vomiting, tachycardia, hypotension and syncope. The cutaneous manifestation is termed urticaria pigmentosa. The skin appearance is a poor guide to the overall systemic involvement. Mast cell degranulation may be precipitated by a number of stimuli, including mechanical irritation, psychological stress, temperature change, alcohol, exercise, bacterial toxins, insect venom, snake venom and certain drugs. These drugs include polymyxin, thiamine, quinine, papaverine, morphine, codeine, atropine, tubocurarine, gallamine, dextran and aspirin. Bone lesions may also occur in these patients, rendering them at risk of pathological fractures.

In the management of these patients any precipitating factors should be avoided (see above). A generous anxiolytic premedication will reduce anxiety and the opportunity should be taken to prescribe an antihistamine. Drugs which are known to readily precipitate the release of histamine should be avoided. No problems have been reported from the use of any of the volatile anaesthetic agents, from suxamethonium or from pethidine. Undue trauma to the skin and mucous membranes (especially the oral and nasal mucosa) should be avoided. It is wise to have ampoules of adrenaline, bronchodilators and antihistamines ready to hand. The patient may be taking steroids, in which case an extra dose of steroid should be considered. Care must be taken in moving and positioning these patients to avoid the occurrence of pathological fractures. Bleeding disorders secondary to the release of heparin from mast cell is possible but rare.

Further reading

Coleman MA, Liberthson RR, Crone RK, Levine FH. *Anesth. Analg.* 1980; **59:** 704–706.
Hosking MP, Warner MA. *Anesth. Analg.* 1987; **66:** 344–346.

Meig's syndrome

Major problems
Reduced respiratory reserve
Intubate for all procedures

The combination of pleural effusion and tumours of the ovary (benign or malignant) makes up Meig's syndrome. The pleural effusion is usually unilateral (right-sided), although it may be bilateral and abdominal ascites might also be present. The effusion is a transudate, low in protein and rapidly re-accumulates after tapping. Rarely, a pericardial effusion may also be present. The patient is often emaciated and anaemic.

The blood count and plasma electrolytes should be checked and brought within acceptable limits pre-operatively. The presence of an effusion and possibly ascites leads to respiratory embarrassment and needs to be drained. If the effusion is not drained then a decrease in ventilatory capacity must be expected. The presence of intra-abdominal ascites raises the intra-abdominal pressure and increases the likelihood of gastro-oesophageal reflux. A rapid sequence anaesthetic induction technique is therefore recommended. Postoperative pulmonary complications are common. Narcotics should be used with care and regular physiotherapy is advisable.

Further reading

Donelly PB. *Anaesthesia,* 1966; **21:** 216−220.

Metastatic myocardial calcification

Metastatic calcific cardiomyopathy

Major problems
Associated cardiomyopathy
Cardiac conduction defects

This condition is the result of a high calcium—phosphate product over a prolonged period of time. It results in the deposition of calcium in the soft tissues; the calcification may appear both in visceral organs (e.g. heart, lungs, kidneys) and in non-visceral tissues (e.g. skin, eyes, subcutaneous tissue). The calcium deposits do not usually show up on X-ray. Calcification in the myocardium is a particular problem and congestive cardiac failure results, which is generally unresponsive to fluid restriction. If calcium is deposited around the AV node or interventricular septum then heart block results.

The principal problem in these patients relates to the associated congestive cardiomyopathy. Myocardial depressant agents (including the volatile anaesthetics) may produce a profound fall in cardiac output and so should be avoided. If heart block is present, it is wise to insert a pacing wire pre-operatively.

Further reading

Bylsma F, Walmsley JBW. *Can. Anaesth. Soc. J.*, 1982; **28**: 167—169.

Methaemoglobinaemia

Major problem
Reduced oxygen carrying capacity

Normal haemoglobin contains iron in the ferrous state. If this iron becomes oxidised to the ferric state oxygen binding is impaired and the oxygen-carrying capacity reduced. The oxyhaemoglobin dissociation curve is progressively shifted towards the left as the methaemoglobin level rises. This oxidised haemoglobin takes on a brownish colour and the patient appears to be cyanosed. It requires a concentration of reduced haemoglobin of greater than 5 g dl^{-1} to give the appearance of cyanosis but only 1.5 g dl^{-1} of methaemoglobin is necessary for the same appearance. Methaemoglobinaemia may be either idiopathic or secondary. In the idiopathic condition there is a congenital absence of the enzyme NADH methaemoglobin reductase which allows methaemoglobin to accumulate. In secondary methaemoglobinaemia methaemoglobin is formed faster than it can be cleared by the enzyme. Drugs which may induce secondary methaemoglobinaemia include lignocaine, prilocaine, benzocaine, nitrites, nitrates, sulphonamides, aniline dyes, and certain antimalarials. It has been reported that sufficient benzocaine can be absorbed from the use of a topical analgesic gel to produce methaemoglobinaemia in small children [1]. The most effective treatment for methaemoglobinaemia is methylene blue (1 mg kg^{-1}). Ascorbic acid and glutathione may also be used.

The presence of methaemoglobinaemia reduces the oxygen carrying capacity of the blood and so should be corrected preoperatively. In patients with idiopathic methaemoglobinaemia drugs which may produce methaemoglobin (see above) should be avoided. There are otherwise no drugs or anaesthetic techniques which are contra-indicated. The development of methaemoglobinaemia will be shown by an incompatibility between the measured values of Pa_{O_2} and Sa_{O_2}. An erroneously low reading for total haemoglobin concentration in a co-oximeter may also be seen. It must be emphasised that methaemoglobinaemia is one of the less common causes of hypoxaemia and is really a diagnosis of exclusion once all other causes have been considered. Methaemoglobin will be seen by pulse oximeters as reduced haemoglobin, resulting in a falsely low displayed saturation. It is likely that the new generation of pulse oximeters will have the facility to introduce a correction for abnormal haemoglobins including methaemoglobin.

Reference

1 Kellett PB, Copeland CS. *Anesthesiology*, 1983; **59**: 463–464.

Further reading

Gabel RA, Bunn HF. *Anesthesiology*, 1974; **40**: 516–518.
Joseph D. *Br. J. Anaesth.*, 1962; **34**: 309–315.
Ohlgisser M, Adler M, Ben-Dov D, Taitelman U, Birkhan HJ, Burzstein S. *Br. J. Anaesth.*, 1978; **50**: 299–301.

Mitral valve prolapse

Major problem
Serious cardiac arrhythmias

Mitral valve prolapse affects about 5–20% of the population, usually in the 20–50 year age group, females more than males. The aetiology is unclear but myxomatous degeneration of the valve cusps, with redundant valve tissue, together with stretching and thinning of the chordae tendineae, has been proposed. The result is to allow prolapse of the mitral valve cusps into the left atrium during systole. An association with certain thoracic skeletal abnormalities has been reported, as has an association with the prolonged QT syndrome. Mitral valve prolapse is usually asymptomatic, although symptoms of fatigue, dyspnoea, palpitations or angina may be present. On auscultation a variable mid-systolic click with a late systolic murmur may be heard. ECG changes may be present (commonly ST and T wave changes) and the diagnosis can be confirmed by echocardiography.

In view of the prevalance of the condition it would seem that the majority of patients with mitral valve prolapse must remain undiagnosed and undergo general anaesthesia without problems. It is unclear why some patients should present problems and others not. There may be a sudden onset of serious cardiac dysrhythmia (ventricular fibrillation is a possibility). The following factors increase the likelihood of dysrhythmias and should be avoided: tachycardia, decreased venous return (e.g. caval compression; high intrathoracic pressure), decreased peripheral vascular resistance, hypotension. The use of certain drugs, including atropine, adrenaline, gallamine and ketamine is inadvisable. Any factors which may increase ventricular irritability, e.g. hypercarbia or electrolyte changes, or which decrease ventricular filling should be avoided. Decreased ventricular filling increases the likelihood of gross valvular prolapse. If a spinal or epidural technique is planned it is important to preload the patient with fluid to prevent hypotension. Antibiotic prophylaxis against bacterial endocarditis should be considered and if the patient is already receiving anti-arrhythmic therapy these drugs must be continued throughout the peri-operative period.

Further reading

Castelhy PA, Dluzneski J, Resurreccion MA, Kleopoulos N, Redko V. *Can. Anaesth. Soc. J.*, 1986; **33**: 795−798.

Forbes RB, Morton GH. *Can. Anaesth. Soc. J.*, 1979; **26**: 424−427.

Kowalski SE. *Can. Anaesth. Soc. J.*, 1985; **32**: 138−141.

Thiagarajah S, Frost EAM. *Anaesthesia*, 1983; **38**: 560−566.

Moya Moya disease

Cerebrovascular Moya Moya disease

Major problem
Avoid hypoglycaemia

This is a rare abnormality of the cerebral circulation where severe stenosis of both the internal carotid arteries is a feature. There is reduced flow through the middle and anterior cerebral arteries and an abnormal network of fine vessels around the basal ganglia. The age groups most affected are 0−7 years and the mid−30s, females more than males. Signs of cerebrovascular insufficiency are common, including generalised or focal motor and sensory disturbances. There may be a history of fits and paroxysmal hemiplegia.

Any technique or treatment which may lead to a decrease in cerebral perfusion must be avoided, including hypocapnia. A general anaesthetic technique using spontaneous respiration is recommended. Whichever technique is chosen the end tidal CO_2 concentration should be monitored to ensure normocapnia or even marginal hypercapnia throughout. The use of a volatile agent with some cerebral vasodilating action, e.g. halothane, may assist in maintaining increased cerebral perfusion.

Further reading

Bingham RM, Wilkinson DJ. *Anaesthesia*, 1985; **40**: 1198−1202.
Sumikawa K, Nagai H. *Anesthesiology*, 1983; **58**: 204−205.

Mucopolysaccharidosis I H
Hurler's syndrome

Major problems
Airway and intubation difficulties
Atlanto-axial instability
Reduced respiratory reserve
Valvular heart lesions

These children have a normal appearance at birth. Deposition of mucopolysaccharide in many tissues, however, leads to a progressive coarsening of the facial features and a deformity of many structures beginning in the first few months of life. They have a large head with coarse lips, large tongue and a relatively small mandible. The teeth are widely separated, the corneas are cloudy, they are short in stature and mentally subnormal. The laryngeal and tracheobronchial cartilages are abnormal. They frequently have kyphotic chests with restricted movement and suffer from recurrent chest infections. Hepatosplenomegaly is common. Coronary artery disease develops at an early age and there may be additional valvular heart disease. Mucopolysaccharidosis I H is inherited in an autosomal recessive fashion and most children die before the age of 10 years from progressive respiratory or cardiac disorders.

These patients present several problems for the anaesthetist. Firstly, the facial features make airway control and intubation difficult. Mucopolysaccharide deposits within the oropharynx, nasopharynx and around the epiglottis are common. Appropriate precautions must therefore be taken for difficulty with airway and intubation. A tracheal tube of a size smaller than expected may be needed and nasal intubation is likely to be impossible due to obstruction of the nose from mucopolysaccharide deposits. If tracheostomy is considered it may be technically very difficult in view of the short, thick neck. Furthermore, instability of the atlanto-axial joint has been reported in these patients. An anti-sialogogue premedication is advisable. The skin and subcutaneous tissues are thickened and this makes venous access difficult. Pre-operative assessment of these patients must include careful appraisal of the cardiac function and reserve because heart failure may be present which must be controlled. Antibiotic prophylaxis may be needed if valvular heart lesions are present. Patients with Hurler's syndrome are particularly prone to chest infections, especially in the postoperative period. Frequent chest physiotherapy is advisable together with humidification of inspired gases and care with the use of all agents which cause respiratory depression. It must be remembered that Hurler's syndrome is a progressive disorder and the older the patient the greater will be the potential problems.

Further reading

Baines D, Keneally J. *Anaesth. Intensive. Care,* 1983; **11**: 198−202.
Kempthorne PM, Brown TCK. *Anaesth. Intensive. Care,* 1983; **11**: 203−207.
King DH, Jones RM, Barnett MB. *Anaesthesia,* 1984; **39**: 126−131.

Mucopolysaccharidosis I S

Scheie's disease

Includes Hurler-Scheie's disease, mucopolysaccharidosis I HS

Major problem
Valvular heart lesions

This disease was previously known as mucopolysaccharidosis V, a category which no longer exists. These patients develop hernias and corneal clouding soon after birth followed by joint stiffness especially of the hands and feet. The other stigmata of mucopolysaccharidosis including thickened skin, gargoyle-like facies, growth retardation and hepatosplenomegaly are all absent. Valvular cardiac lesions frequently develop, in particular aortic regurgitation. These patients usually have normal stature, intelligence and life span.

The subgroup, mucopolysaccharidosis I HS (Hurler-Scheie's disease) appears to be an intermediate between types I H (see page 155) and I S. Some coarsening of the facial features is seen and they are usually mentally subnormal.

Patients with mucopolysaccharidosis I S or I HS do not usually present a great problem to the anaesthetist. Care should be taken, however, in positioning the patients because of their stiff joints. Careful pre-operative evaluation of the cardiac status is important and antibiotic prophylaxis against bacterial endocarditis should be considered if appropriate.

Further reading

Baines D, Keneally J. *Anaesth. Intensive. Care,* 1983; **11**: 198−202.
Kempthorne PM, Brown TCK. *Anaesth. Intensive. Care,* 1983; **11**: 203−207.
King DH, Jones RM, Barnett MB. *Anaesthesia,* 1984; **39**: 126−131.

Mucopolysaccharidosis II

Hunter's disease

Major problems
Valvular heart lesions with heart failure
Airway and intubation difficulties

These patients appear normal at birth. Coarsening of facial features begins at about two years of age. Thickening of the lips, tongue and nostrils occurs, together with growth retardation, joint stiffness and hepatosplenomegaly. Chest deformity is present with pectus excavatum and occasionally kyphoscoliosis. The presence of lymphoid tissue in the larynx results in noisy breathing with partial upper airway obstruction. Early onset coronary artery disease is present together with valvular heart lesions, and heart failure is often the end result. The patients are usually of normal intelligence and do not have clouding of the corneas. Hunter's disease is inherited in an X-linked recessive manner, and therefore only affects males.

The cardiac status must be carefully assessed pre-operatively and any heart failure brought under control. Antibiotic prophylaxis should be considered if valvular lesions are present. Care must be taken in positioning these patients due to the stiff joints. The presence of partial upper airway obstruction may make for difficulties in airway management and tracheal intubation, and appropriate precautions should be taken. With these exceptions there are no reported specific contra-indications to any anaesthetic drug or technique.

Further reading

Baines D, Keneally J. *Anaesth. Intensive. Care,* 1983; **11:** 198–202.
Kempthorne PM, Brown TCK. *Anaesth. Intensive Care,* 1983; **11:** 203–207.
King DH, Jones RM, Barnett MB. *Anaesthesia,* 1984; **39:** 126–131.

Mucopolysaccharidosis III

Sanfilippo syndrome

Major problems
None

This disorder is the mildest of the mucopolysaccharidoses. The children have normal appearance at birth and initially grow and develop normally. Development begins to slow, however, as childhood advances and there is a steady decline in mental development leading to frank dementia in late childhood. Emotional disturbances and agitation are common. Unlike the other mucopolysacchariodoses there are no cardiac or skeletal problems or hepatosplenomegaly. There may be minimal coarsening of facial features.

No anaesthetic problems have been described in these patients.

Further reading

Baines D, Keneally J. *Anaesth. Intensive. Care*, 1983; **11**: 198−202.
Kempthorne PM, Brown TCK. *Anaesth. Intensive. Care*, 1983; **11**: 203−207.
King DH, Jones RM, Barnett MB. *Anaesthesia*, 1984; **39**: 126−131.

Mucopolysaccharidosis IV

Morquio's syndrome, chondro-osteodystrophy

Major problems
Atlanto-axial instability
Diminished respiratory reserve
Airway and intubation difficulties

Patients with this autosomal recessive inherited disorder are severely dwarfed with short trunk and limbs, lax joints and a marked kyphosis. The distortion of the chest leads to respiratory impairment and the patients usually do not survive beyond 30 years of age. Facial appearances include a short nose with prominent maxilla and widely spaced teeth with defective enamel. Corneal opacities and hearing disorders are common although intellectual development is usually normal. The heart is usually involved with valvular lesions, in particular aortic incompetence. Defective cartilage in the neck results in atlanto-axial instability.

It is essential to assess carefully the patient's respiratory and cardiovascular systems before anaesthesia. Chest movement and cardiac function may be severely limited. Antibiotic prophylaxis against bacterial endocarditis should be considered. Great care must be taken with movement and positioning of the patient, in particular the neck, due to the likelihood of atlanto-axial instability. The use of a neck-brace or a plaster cast has been recommended. The combination of neck problems and facial deformities results in airway and intubation difficulties. All appropriate precautions for the difficult intubation must therefore be taken before beginning. Muscle relaxants must be avoided until the trachea has been intubated. Drugs which are myocardial depressants or respiratory depressants should be given with care and in reduced dosage. Respiratory problems are common during the postoperative period and aggressive chest physiotherapy may be required.

Further reading

Baines D, Keneally J. *Anaesth. Intensive Care*, 1983; **11:** 198–202.
Birkinshaw KJ. *Anaesthesia*, 1975; **30:** 46–49.
Jones AEP, Croley TF. *Anesthesiology*, 1979; **51:** 261–262.
Kempthorne PM, Brown TCK. *Anaesth. Intensive Care*, 1983; **11:** 203–207.
King DH, Jones RM, Barnett MB. *Anaesthesia*, 1984; **39:** 126–131.

Mucopolysaccharidosis VI

Maroteaux-Lamy syndrome

Major problems
Airway and intubation difficulties
Possible atlanto-axial instability

These patients appear normal at birth then slowly develop coarsening of facial features, kyphoscoliosis and growth retardation. They are usually of normal intelligence. Some patients have a degree of atlanto-axial instability and care must therefore be taken with neck movements. They suffer repeated chest infections which result in chronic respiratory problems. Hepatosplenomegaly, anaemia and thrombocytopenia are not uncommon and the patients usually die from cardiorespiratory failure by the age of 20 years.

The respiratory and cardiovascular systems must be assessed pre-operatively. It is wise also to check the coagulation status. The facial features and neck instability may lead to difficulties in maintaining the airway and with intubation. Appropriate precautions for a difficult intubation must be made before starting anaesthesia. Drugs which are myocardial depressants or respiratory depressants should be administered with care.

Further reading

Baines D, Keneally J. *Anaesth. Intensive Care*, 1983; **11:** 198−202.
Kempthorne PM, Brown TCK. *Anaesth. Intensive Care*, 1983; **11:** 203−207.
King DH, Jones RM, Barnett MB. *Anaesthesia*, 1984; **39:** 126−131.

Multiple sclerosis

Disseminated sclerosis, demyelinating disorders

Major problems
None

Abnormalities of myelination lead to the formation of sclerotic plaques in the central nervous system with subsequent patchy demyelination. The exact symptoms and signs depend upon the site of the plaques. It is a disease of young adults who present with motor weakness, visual symptoms, sensory symptoms, and paraesthesia. There are remissions and relapses superimposed on a slowly progressive overall deterioration. It is a disease of temperate climates and is rare in members of the Asian and African races. Stress and an increase in body temperature often precipitate a relapse. The aetiology is unclear and there is presently no specific curative treatment.

Pre-operatively the history, progression and extent of the disease should be determined. Patients may range from being almost unaffected to being totally bedridden. The patient should be asked about any history of fits, the incidence of which is increased. A neurological examination is advisable. The patient may be taking ACTH or steroid therapy, in which case perioperative steroid cover will be necessary. There are no particular anaesthetic or sedative agents which are contra-indicated in this condition. Unless there is a positive history of epilepsy enflurane, methohexitone and possibly propofol are contra-indicated. Anticholinergic agents should be avoided as their use tends to result in a small increase in body temperature. The nondepolarising muscle relaxants may safely be used although increased sensitivity may be encountered and so dosage should be reduced. It is wise to avoid suxamethonium if possible because reports have described hyperkalaemia (there may be denervated muscle present) and also myotonia, this leads to a rise in body temperature. Body temperature should be monitored throughout to allow any rise to be detected and treated early. A small fall in body temperature does not matter and may even be beneficial. Autonomic instability results in labile blood pressure, and so hypotension when changing position under anaesthesia is likely. Suggestions have been made that a relapse in the condition may follow anaesthesia or surgery. However, there is no good evidence to incriminate either surgery or anaesthesia directly. Stress or pyrexia (not uncommon in the postoperative period) may precipitate a relapse. An increase in platelet adhesiveness has been reported and the use of prophylaxis against DVT would therefore seem to be advisable.

The use of local or regional blocks in these patients is controversial. There is no good evidence to link any of these techniques with changes in the course of the disease. Spinal anaesthesia has been used successfully in these patients. In view of the chronic progressive course of the condition, however, many people feel it wise to avoid these techniques.

Further reading

Azar I. *Anesthesiology*, 1984; **61:** 173–187.
Beavis RE, Davies MJ. *Anaesthesia*, 1986; **41:** 1258–1259.
Berger JM, Ontell R. *Anesthesiology*, 1987; **66:** 400–405.
Jones RM, Healy TEJ. *Anaesthesia*, 1980; **35:** 879–884.
Siemkowitz E. *Anaesthesia*, 1976; **31:** 1211–1216.

Muscular dystrophy

Duchenne muscular dystrophy,
progressive muscular dystrophy,
pseudohypertrophic muscular dystrophy

Major problems
Reduced respiratory reserve
Cardiomyopathy, tachycardia, heart failure
Acute gastric dilatation
Avoid suxamethonium
Possible association with malignant hyperpyrexia

This degenerative disease of skeletal muscle is inherited in an X-linked recessive manner and therefore found only in males, with an incidence of $25-30:100\,000$. Slowly developing weakness makes the patient wheelchair bound by the early teens. Later in the disease process the myocardium becomes involved and tachycardia may occur spontaneously or secondary to excitement. Kyphoscoliosis also develops and patients usually die of cardiac or respiratory failure by age 20. Characteristic changes have been described in the ECG of patients with Duchenne muscular dystrophy, namely a tall R wave in lead V1 and deep Q waves in leads V4—V6 [1].

Suxamethonium must be avoided [2] because hyperkalaemia, cardiac dysrhythmias, myoglobinuria, rhabdomyolysis, and renal failure may result. An increased incidence of malignant hyperpyrexia has been reported in these patients [3, 4]; the temperature should be monitored throughout. Lower doses than usual of nondepolarising muscle relaxants have been found to be effective and atracurium has been recommended. Halothane is best avoided because it has been known to induce malignant hyperpyrexia in patients with Duchenne muscular dystrophy and also cardiomyopathy may be present. Atropine produces a tachycardia which may be a problem. Respiratory depressant agents should be used with care in view of the increased sensitivity of these patients to these drugs. Lung function is impaired, and so pre-operative pulmonary function tests should be performed.

Chest physiotherapy will be needed postoperatively and a period of controlled ventilation may be necessary.

Acute gastric dilatation is not uncommon [5] due probably to changes in smooth muscle which are similar to those in striated muscle. Gastric emptying may be slower than usual [6]. Correction of electrolyte imbalance, avoidance of oral fluids for 48 hours post-operation and avoiding the supine position may lessen the risk of gastric dilatation. If orthopaedic procedures make the supine position necessary, then a nasogastric tube should be passed and the stomach drained continuously.

References

1 Slucka C. *Circulation*, 1986; **38:** 933—939.
2 Milne B, Rosales JK. *Can. Anaesth. Soc. J.*, 1982, **29:** 250—254.
3 Wang JM, Stanley TH. *Can. Anaesth. Soc. J.*, 1986, **33:** 492—497.
4 Brownell AKW, Paasuke RT, Elash A, Fowlow SB, Seagram CGF, Diewold RJ, Friesen C. *Anesthesiology*, 1983, **58:** 180—182.
5 Wislicki L. *Anaesthesia*, 1962; **17:** 482—487.
6 Smith CL, Bush GH. *Br. J. Anaesth.*, 1985, **57:** 1113—1118.

Further reading

Henderson WAV. *Can. Anaesth. Soc. J.*, 1984, **31:** 444.
Miller ED, Sanders DB, Rowlingson JC, Berry FA, Sussman MD, Epstein RM. *Anesthesiology*, 1978, **48:** 146—148.

Myasthenia gravis
Myasthenia congenita, congenital myasthenia gravis,
neonatal myasthenia gravis

Major problems
Sensitive to nondepolarising muscle relaxants
Unpredictable response to depolarising relaxants

This autoimmune disorder of the neuromuscular junction results in increased weakness and fatigability. The mainstay of treatment is anticholinergic therapy and patients often require to remain on this treatment for life. Thymectomy occasionally affords some reduction in symptoms. Females are affected more often than males; the disease usually begins in early adulthood but may appear at any age. Neonatal myasthenia gravis appears in 20−30% of babies born to myasthenic mothers and is only temporary.

The principal feature of patients with myasthenia gravis is an abnormal response to neuromuscular blocking agents. The patients are extremely sensitive to nondepolarising muscle relaxants; a neuromuscular blockade of greater than 90% may be produced by doses as small as 5 mg of tubocurarine, 0.5 mg of pancuronium or 3 mg of atracurium. The response to suxamethonium is less predictable and a phase two block appears very early. It is recommended that anticholinesterase therapy is stopped 12−24 hours pre-operatively. The patients are then beginning to become weak and the use of a volatile agent will reduce neuromuscular transmission further allowing sufficient flaccidity for most surgical procedures to be performed. If a more profound block is required then tiny doses of a nondepolarising relaxant should be administered. Reports have suggested that atracurium is at present the drug of choice [1, 2]. At the termination of surgery the administration of neostigmine should increase muscle power again. It is not uncommon to require a short period of controlled ventilation in the postoperative period and even if not, the patient should be observed postoperatively on a high dependency nursing unit. Myasthenic symptoms may

168

be made worse by a number of other drugs, including procaina-

be made worse by a number of other drugs, including procaina-

mothers may be weak and require a period of controlled venti-

lation. They should in any case be carefully observed for several

References

References

1 Baraka A, Dajani A. *Anesth. Analg.*, 1984; **63:** 1127–1130.
2 Hunter JM. *Br. J. Anaesth.*, 1986; **58:** 89S.
3 Rolbin SH, Levinson G, Schnider SM, Wright RG. *Anesth. Analg.*, 1978; **57:** 441–447.

Further reading

Azar I. *Anesthesiology*, 1984; **61:** 173–187.
Dalal FY, Bennett EJ, Gegg WS. *Anaesthesia*, 1972; **27:** 61–65.
Davies DW, Steward DG. *Can. Anaesth. Soc. J.*, 1973; **20:** 253–258.
Foldes FF, McNall PG. *Anesthesiology*, 1962; **23:** 837–872.
Girnar DS, Weinreich AI. *Anesth. Analg.*, 1976; **55:** 13–17.
Secher O. *Acta Anaesth. Scand.*, 1967; **11:** 245–259.

Myasthenic syndrome

Eaton-Lambert syndrome, pseudomyasthenia

Major problems
Increased sensitivity to muscle relaxants
Poor response to anticholinergic agents

The association of weakness and ready fatigability in association with an underlying malignancy is the myasthenic syndrome. Unlike myasthenia gravis, there is an increase in muscular strength on exercise and patients frequently complain of aching pains in the limbs. There is a poor response to anticholinergics but guanidine, 4-aminopyridine and calcium may decrease the weakness.

These patients are exquisitely sensitive to muscle relaxants: 5 mg of tubocurarine lasted for 24 hours in one patient [1]. It is advisable to avoid relaxants totally if at all possible. Anti-tumour agents may be administered to the patient because of the underlying malignancy and these may exacerbate the problem. A prolonged response to pancuronium has been reported when a patient was given a dose of an alkylating agent [2]. These patients are very likely to require a period of controlled ventilation postoperatively followed by high dependency nursing.

References

1 Wise RP. *Br. J. Anaesth.*, 1962; **17**: 488–504.
2 Bennett EJ, Schmidt GB, Patel HP, Grundy EM. *Anesthesiology*, 1976; **46**: 220–221.

Further reading

Agoston S, Van Weerden T, Westra P, Brockert A. *Br. J. Anaesth.*, 1978; **50**: 383–385.
Azar I. *Anesthesiology*, 1984; **61**: 173–187.
Clements JG. *Anesthesiology*, 1977; **47**: 317.

169

Myopathy — carnitine deficiency

Major problem
Avoid hypoglycaemia

This disorder is inherited in an autosomal recessive manner. There is accumulation of lipid within the fibres of skeletal muscle and muscle carnitine levels are reduced to 10−20% of normal. Clinically there is a slowly progressive myopathy commonly affecting the muscles of the face, neck and pharynx. There are two types of this disease, the myopathic form and the systemic form. Muscular weakness is common to both but the liver is also involved in the systemic form with hepatic encephalopathy a frequent cause of death. Cardiomyopathy is also common. Treatment with carnitine and steroids may improve the symptoms.

There is only one report of anaesthesia in this conditon [1]. The child suffered from frequent recurrent episodes of pneumonia. An uneventful anaesthetic was administered using just nitrous oxide, oxygen and halothane. A dextrose intravenous infusion was established before anaesthesia and maintained throughout the peri-operative period because the tissues are more dependent upon glucose as an energy source in carnitine deficiency.

Reference

1 Beilin B, Shulman D, Schiffman Y. *Anaesthesia,* 1986; **41:** 92.

Myotonia congenita

Thomsen's disease

Major problem

Suxamethonium is contra-indicated

This condition is inherited in an autosomal dominant manner and is less common than myotonica dystrophia. Myotonia is a prominent feature and is more marked than in myotonica dystrophia although the disease runs a more benign course overall. Myotonia is classically more severe after rest and is relieved by exercise. It may also be exacerbated by cold. There is a diffuse hypertrophy of muscles which show no dystrophic changes. Cardiac and smooth muscles are rarely involved.

Anaesthetic considerations are similar to those for myotonica dystrophia [1]. These patients are sensitive to barbiturates, opiates and other respiratory depressant agents. Suxamethonium is contra-indicated because it is likely to initiate a myotonic episode; the nondepolarising relaxants are safe. Anticholinesterases should also be avoided because their effects are unpredictable and a myotonic episode may result. Local anaesthetic agents may safely be used. Myotonic episodes may respond to quinidine or to the direct injection of local anaesthetic into the muscle. Postoperative respiratory depression may be a problem and a period of controlled ventilation may be needed together with physiotherapy. There is a reported association with malignant hyperpyrexia [2, 3].

References

1 Ellis FR. *Br. J. Anaesth.*, 1974; **46**: 603–612.
2 King JO, Denborough MA, Zapt PW. *Lancet*, 1972; **1**: 365–370.
3 Saidman LJ, Havard ES, Eger EI. *J.A.M.A.*, 1964; **190**: 1029–1032.

Myotonica dystrophia (adult type)

Dystrophia myotonica, myotonic dystrophy,
myotonia atrophica, Steinart's disease,
Hoffman's disease

Major problems
Sensitivity to respiratory depressants
Avoid suxamethonium
Avoid anticholinesterases
Dysrythmias

This disorder is inherited in an autosomal dominant manner and usually becomes evident in the third and fourth decades. Variable expressivity results in a range of grades of severity from patients who are almost unaffected to those who are wheelchair bound. The functional problem is that of muscle weakness and wasting which is associated with myotonia. It is a progressive condition and develops into a multisystem disease which also affects smooth muscle and cardiac muscle. Myotonia develops on contraction of muscles and the classic presentation is that of a patient who, having shaken hands, cannot let go. Other characteristics include frontal baldness, gonadal atrophy, cataracts, cardiomyopathy, ECG conduction disorders and a low IQ.

Pre-operatively, ECG and lung function tests should be performed as part of the regular anaesthetic assessment. These patients are very sensitive to thiopentone, opiates and other respiratory depressants and a period of postoperative controlled ventilation may be necessary until the depressant effect has worn off [1, 2]. Volatile anaesthetic agents are safe although their use may be followed by postoperative shivering which itself may induce a myotonic episode. Suxamethonium causes a myotonic reaction and also hyperkalaemia and is therefore contraindicated. The nondepolarising muscle relaxants are safe, although they will not affect myotonic spasm because it is the result of a muscle phenomenon distal to the neuromuscular junction. The response to anticholinesterases is unpredictable—neuromuscular blockade may or may not be satisfactorily reversed and a myo-

172

tonic episode may result. It may be advisable therefore to use one of the newer shorter acting muscle relaxants and to await spontaneous recovery [3, 4]. Over 50% of these patients have associated cardiomyopathy. It is wise to administer agents which are myocardial depressants (including halothane) with care. This, together with cardiac conduction defects, may lead to sudden cardiac arrest at any time [1]. The smooth muscle of the gastrointestinal tract may be affected, resulting in a reduced rate of gastric emptying. This together with disorders of swallowing, puts these patients at an increased risk of vomiting, regurgitation and aspiration [5, 6]. Pregnancy often makes the symptoms of myotonica dystrophia worse [7].

Local anaesthetic agents may be safely used [7, 8]. They will only reduce myotonic spasms, however, when injected directly into affected muscle. A problem with postpartum haemorrhage due to dystonic uterine contractions was successfully treated by the topical application of bupivacaine to the uterine muscle [7]. The use of dantrolene was examined in one case; the results were inconclusive [9].

Postoperatively, these patients have a weak cough and shallow weak respirations. Physiotherapy and a period of controlled ventilation may be necessary.

References

1 Aldridge L. *Br. J. Anaesth.*, 1985; **57:** 1119−1130.
2 Mitchell MM, Ali HH, Savarese JJ. *Anesthesiology*, 1978; **49:** 44−48.
3 Nightingale P, Healy TEJ, McGuiness K. *Br. J. Anaesth.*, 1975; **57:** 1131−1135.
4 Stirt JA, Stone DJ, Weinberg G, Willson DF, Sternick CS, Sussman MD. *Anesth. Analg.*, 1985; **64:** 369−370.
5 Ishizawa Y, Yamaguchi H, Dohi S, Koyama K. *Anesth. Analg.*, 1986; **65:** 1066−1068.
6 Paterson RA, Tousignant M, Skene DS. *Can. Anaesth. Soc. J.*, 1985; **32:** 418−421.
7 Cope DK, Miller JN. *Anesth. Analg.*, 1986; **65:** 687−690.
8 Wheeler AS, James FM. *Anesthesiology*, 1979; **50:** 169.
9 Phillips DC, Ellis FR, Exley KA, Ness MA. *Anaesthesia*, 1984; **39:** 568−573.

Myotonica dystrophia (congenital)

Major problems
Respiratory insufficiency
Avoid suxamethonium

Neonates present with generalised hypotonia, facial diplegia, and a 'tent-shaped' mouth. Approximately 50% also have talipes equinovarus. There may be difficulties with sucking and swallowing. Both babies described required prolonged respiratory support. Respiratory insufficiency is common and may be due to a lack of central respiratory drive or due to the muscle disease itself. Myotonia does not usually appear until about 10 years of age. The disorder is inherited in an autosomal dominant manner and the mother is commonly the carrier.

It is wise to avoid respiratory depressants. If general anaesthesia is necessary drugs which are myocardial depressants should be avoided. Halothane caused profound hypotension in one patient [1]. Depolarising muscle relaxants should be avoided because of the likelihood of producing a contracture of the muscles. It is likely that a period of postoperative respiratory support will be needed. A regional technique should be considered. A caudal block was used to good effect in a two-year-old child with this condition [2].

References

1 Bray RJ, Inkster JS. *Anaesthesia,* 1984; **39:** 1007—1011.
2 Alexander C, Wolf S, Ghia JN. *Anesthesiology,* 1981; **55:** 597—598.

Nemaline myopathy

Major problems
Restrictive lung disorder
Possible intubation difficulties
Abnormal response to suxamethonium

This congenital myopathy is inherited in an autosomal dominant fashion. All skeletal muscles, including the diaphragm, are affected with a symmetrical weakness. Patients usually present in the newborn period with hypotonia, weakness and poor sucking. Subsequent development is delayed. Skeletal deformities including kyphosis, scoliosis and pectus excavatum are common. Smooth muscle and cardiac muscle are not usually involved. There may be facial abnormalities, including a narrow face with a high arched palate and micrognathia. The disorder is usually nonprogressive and does not interfere with normal life expectancy. More severe progressive forms have been described.

There are several considerations regarding anaesthesia in these patients [1]. Pre-operative assessment should include an examination of the mouth and airway. It is wise to make appropriate preparations in case difficulties are encountered with intubation. Pulmonary function tests should also be performed before anaesthesia. A restrictive lung disorder is common and in longstanding cases pulmonary hypertension may be present. There may also be an abnormality of central respiratory control which will make the patient sensitive to barbiturates, opiates and other respiratory depressants. Theoretically, the use of depolarising muscle relaxants is inadvisable in patients with a myopathy. There is one case report where suxamethonium was used and the drug had an abnormally slow onset of effect and did not produce complete neuromuscular blockade [2]. The response to pancuronium was normal.

References

1 Cunliffe M, Burrows FA. *Can. Anaesth. Soc. J.*, 1985; **32:** 543−547.
2 Heard SO, Kaplan RF. *Anesthesiology*, 1983; **59:** 588−590.

Neurofibromatosis

Von Recklinghausen's disease

Major problems
Possible airway/intubation difficulties
Unpredictable response to muscle relaxants

Von Recklinghausen's neurofibromatosis is inherited in an autosomal dominant manner. It is characterised by multiple tumours, originating in nerve trunks, which may affect almost any organ of the body. Café au lait spots are also present on the skin. Clinical features are many and varied. Central nervous system involvement is common, with an increased incidence of meningiomas and gliomas as well as neurofibromas in the brain and spinal cord. The presence of bulky neurofibromas may cause problems if they occur in the mouth or airway, within the lumen of the heart or close to joints. Other associations include mental retardation, kyphoscoliosis, phaeochromocytoma (about 1%), lung cysts, renal artery dysplasia with hypertension and bone cysts. It is a progressive condition and problems may therefore increase with age.

Pre-operative assessment of the airway, including mouth opening and neck mobility is important. A neurofibroma within the mouth or on the tongue may make airway control and intubation very difficult [1]. Lung function tests are advisable, particularly if there is kyphoscoliosis or known lung pathology. In view of the known association with phaeochromocytoma it is wise to maintain a high index of suspicion for this condition and to screen pre-operatively if indicated. There are no particular anaesthetic agents or techniques which are contra-indicated. Sensitivity has been reported in several patients to nondepolarising muscle relaxants and a varied response to suxamethonium [2–6]. It is advisable therefore to initially administer a reduced dose and to monitor the effect. Regional blocks, including spinals and epidurals, are not contra-indicated and have been used successfully, although co-existing kyphoscoliosis may give rise to difficulties in performing the block and the spread of anaesthesia may be unpredictable [7]. A case has been reported [8] where a mobile, pedunculated lesion within the cranium, close to to the base of the brain, shifted position on turning the patient prone, leading to sudden bradycardia followed by neurogenic pulmonary oedema.

References

1 Crozier WC. *Anaesthesia*, 1987; **42:** 1209−1211.
2 Manser J. *Br. J. Anaesth.*, 1970; **42:** 183.
3 Yamashita M, Matsuki A. *Br. J. Anaesth.*, 1975; **47:** 1032.
4 Nagao H, Yamashita M, Shinozaki Y, Oyama T. *Br. J. Anaesth.*, 1983; **55:** 253.
5 Baraka A. *Br. J. Anaesth.*, 1974; **46:** 701−703.
6 Magbagbeola JAO. *Br. J. Anaesth.*, 1970; **42:** 710.
7 Fisher MMcD. *Anaesthesia*, 1975; **30:** 648−650.
8 Van Aken H, Scherer R, Lawin P. *Anaesthesia*, 1987; **37:** 827−829.

Obesity

Morbid obesity

Major problems
Difficult airway and intubation
Inability to lie flat
Venous access problems
Increased incidence of deep venous thrombosis,
 tracheal aspiration and postoperative
 respiratory problems

A person is generally regarded as obese when their weight is greater than 10% above the ideal predicted weight for their height and morbidly obese when their weight is more than twice that ideal. Anaesthetic problems are many in the obese patient and tend to increase with the degree of obesity and duration of time that the patient has been overweight. If the condition is secondary to an endocrinological or metabolic disorder, consideration should also be given to the underlying pathology. There are reports of sudden unexpected deaths during anaesthesia in morbidly obese patients.

The thick layer of fat on the chest wall and abdomen results in a decrease in chest wall compliance, total lung capacity and functional residual capacity (FRC). There is premature airway closure. These problems are accentuated by the supine position and render many patients incapable of lying flat. The work of respiration is increased with a raised oxygen consumption, a raised carbon dioxide output and increased resting alveolar ventilation [1, 2]. A number of these patients suffer from sleep apnoeas or primary alveolar hypoventilation (see page 20). The total blood volume and cardiac output are increased and many of these patients are hypertensive. Pulmonary hypertension is not uncommon and there is an increase in cardiac workload and an increased incidence of ischaemic heart disease [1, 2]. The incidence of deep venous thrombosis is high in these patients.

Pre-operative assessment should include pulmonary function tests and measurement of arterial blood gases. Any sedative premedicant should be prescribed with caution. The chest X-ray may be difficult to interpret. Prophylaxis against deep venous thrombosis should be considered. In view of the greater difficulty involved in the lifting and positioning of these patients, it is helpful to ask the patient to position himself before the induction of anaesthesia if this is practical. The prone and Trendelenburg positions should be avoided. Preoxygenation should be undertaken but the reduced FRC holds less oxygen than might be otherwise expected. The combination of a high intra-abdominal pressure and a hiatus hernia (common in obese patients) increases the likelihood of the regurgitation of gastric contents and pretreatment with H_2 receptor antagonists, antacids and metoclopramide has been recommended, together with cricoid pressure [3]. Intravenous access is often difficult and intramuscular injections may be almost impossible. Doses of drugs are difficult to predict because, although fat people require greater quantities of drugs than is usual, their overall requirement on a body weight basis is less. Laryngoscopy and intubation may be difficult due to the enlarged fat pads around the face, neck and airway; awake intubation under local anaesthesia has been recommended [4]. Maintenance of the airway using a face-mask may also be difficult. For all but the most minor procedures a technique including tracheal intubation and controlled ventilation is advisable. High inflation pressures may be needed but care should be taken to keep these as low as possible because the higher the inflation pressure, the greater will be the reduction in pulmonary blood flow. In one report a sterile rod was passed through the abdominal panniculus and this was then raised with a hydraulic lift to reduce pressure on the abdomen [4]. The uptake of lipid soluble anaesthetic agents into fat depots is considerable and this will delay recovery; the use of propofol has been recommended [5].

Monitoring the blood pressure can be difficult due to errors when using an external cuff on a fat arm. The insertion of an indwelling arterial line may be necessary, a technique which also allows repeated blood gas measurements to be made more easily.

In the postoperative period the patient should be nursed in a semi-recumbent posture in order to assist ventilation [6]. Supplemental oxygen should be given for at least 24 hours. Pulmonary complications are frequent, particularly following abdominal surgery. Postoperative analgesia must be prescribed with care so as to avoid undue respiratory depression. Thoracic epidurals have been used to good advantage [7].

Regional nerve blocks, including spinals and epidurals, may be used but they are technically difficult to perform and may require a long (15 cm) needle. The landmarks of the back are easier to locate with the patient in the sitting position. A reduced dose of local analgesic agent should be used in the epidural space [8]. The subsequent position required for surgery must be considered because the patient may find it impossible to lie flat.

References

1 Ramsey-Stewart G. *Anaesthesia,* 1985; **13:** 399–406.
2 Tsueda K, Debrand M, Zeok SS, Wright BD, Griffin WO. *Anesth. Analg.,* 1979; **58:** 345–349.
3 Manchikanti L, Roush JR, Colliver JA. *Anesth. Analg.,* 1986; **65:** 195–199.
4 Wyner J, Brodsky JB, Merrill RC. *Anesth. Analg.,* 1981; **60:** 691–693.
5 Kirby IJ, Howard EC. *Anaesthesia,* 1987; **42:** 1125–1128.
6 Vaughan RW, Bauer S, Wise L. *Anesth. Analg.,* 1976; **55:** 37–41.
7 Buckley FP, Robinson NB, Simonowitz DA, Dellinger EP. *Anaesthesia,* 1983; **38:** 840–851.
8 Hodgkinson R, Husain FJ. *Anesth. Analg.,* 1980; **59:** 89–92.

Occipital encephalocoele

Major problems
Defective thermoregulation
Possible difficult intubation

This uncommon congenital defect presents at birth. There is herniation of the occipital lobes of the brain through a bony defect and urgent surgery is usually necessary in the neonatal period. It is likely that there are additional extensive malformations present within the brain and the base of the skull. There is an association with hydrocephalus, the Klippel-Feil syndrome (see page 128) and cleft lip and palate. Disturbances in central autonomic regulation are present, in particular defects in thermoregulation.

The position of the lesion means that the patient cannot lie supine without careful arrangements of pillows and supports. Intubation may be difficult and may have to be performed with the child in the lateral position. In view of the immature thermoregulatory system body temperature is more labile than normal and so great care must be taken to conserve heat.

Further reading

Creighton RE, Relton JES, Meridy HW. *Can. Anaesth. Soc. J.,* 1974; **21**: 403–405.

Ocular muscular dystrophy

Ocular myopathy

Major problem
Increased sensitivity to nondepolarising relaxants

This syndrome is characterised by progressive external ophthal-moplegia, ptosis and limb and trunk weakness. It is inherited in an autosomal dominant manner and possesses features similar both to other muscular dystrophies and to myasthenia gravis.

The feature of most importance to anaesthetists is the extreme sensitivity to nondepolarising neuromuscular blocking agents. The response to anticholinesterases is also abnormal and there is no improvement in symptoms on reversal of neuromuscular blockade following the administration of an anticholinesterase. In the case report cited, the response to suxamethonium was normal [1]. A further general anaesthetic was then given using halothane without problems.

Reference

1 Robertson JA. *Anaesthesia,* 1984; **39:** 251−253.

Oculo-auriculovertebral dysplasia

Goldenhars syndrome

Major problems
Difficult airway
Difficult intubation
Congenital heart disease

The abnormalities in this syndrome are mainly confined to the head and neck. The patients have a variety of eye and ear abnormalities in addition to micrognathia, maxillary or mandibular hypoplasia and cleft or high arched palate [1]. Disorders of the cervical vertebrae may result in limited movement of the neck. Twenty per cent of patients have an associated congenital heart disease. The disorder is not inherited but probably arises due to a vascular abnormality during embryological development of the first and second arches. Both male and females are equally affected.

The major problem facing the anaesthetist is one of airway management. The patient will be difficult or even impossible to intubate and the external appearance is not a reliable guide to potential problems [2]. All aids to intubation should be prepared. One case report [3] describes the satisfactory use of a retrograde technique for intubation. The use of an elective tracheostomy under local anaesthesia has also been recommended. It is wise to have a surgeon standing by to perform an urgent tracheostomy if necessary. The airway problems must not direct attention away from other systems. The possibility of congenital heart disease must also be borne in mind. Pre-operative assessment of cardiac function is important in these patients and if any abnormality is present antibiotic prophylaxis against bacterial endocarditis must be considered.

References

1 Feingold M, Baum J. *Am. J. Dis. Child.*, 1978; **132:** 136–138.
2 Stehling L. *Am. J. Dis. Child.*, 1978; **132:** 878.
3 Cooper CMS, Murray-Wilson A. *Anaesthesia*, 1987; **42:** 1198–1200.

Further reading

Scholtes JL, Veyckemans F, Van Obbergh L, Verellen G, Gribomont BF. *Anaesth. Intensive Care*, 1987; **15:** 338–340.

Ophthalmoplegia plus

Progressive ophthalmoplegia,
progressive external ophthalmoplegia,
Kearns Sayer syndrome

Major problems
Possible atrio-ventricular conduction block
Sensitive to anaesthetic induction agents

Patients with this disorder have bilateral ptosis, weakness of the external ocular muscles and pigmented retinopathy. Divergent squint, diplopia and blurred vision are common symptoms. In addition there may be weakness of certain proximal limb muscles (e.g. shoulder girdle) and unusual cardiac conduction defects making the patients prone to the sudden onset of complete heart block. If this latter problem is prevented by an indwelling pacemaker then they should have a normal life span.

There have been three case reports of anaesthesia for patients with ophthalmoplegia plus. In two of these, patients were reported to be very sensitive to anaesthetic induction agents (4 mg of etomidate in a 76 kg patient [1] and 75 mg of thiopentone in a 56 kg patient [2]). In the third a normal induction dose of thiamylal 4 mg kg^{-1} was used without problem. No difficulties were encountered with the use of suxamethonium, pancuronium, neostigmine, atropine, hyoscine, levorphanol, pethidine, fentanyl, halothane or nitrous oxide. It would therefore appear that, apart from a possible reduced requirement for induction agents, no specific anaesthetic drugs or techniques are contraindicated. In view of the likelihood of the sudden development of complete heart block it would be wise to have equipment for the rapid insertion of an external pacing wire readily to hand.

References

1 James RH. *Anaesthesia,* 1986; **41:** 216.
2 James RH. *Anaesthesia,* 1986; **40:** 88.

Further reading

D'Ambra MN, Dedrick D, Savarese JJ. *Anesthesiology,* 1979; **51:** 343−345.

Opitz Frias syndrome

Hypospadias-dysphagia syndrome,
G-syndrome

Major problem
Recurrent tracheal aspiration

This rare congenital syndrome affects males principally but a milder form may appear in females. The syndrome is complex. Facial features may include short palpebral fissures with an upward slant and upper epicanthic fold, anteversion of nostrils, prominent lateral skull ridges, high arched palate and micrognathia. A disorder of oespophageal motility leads to dysphagia with recurrent tracheal aspiration. The child has a hoarse weak cry and may have stridor due to an immature larynx. The genital abnormalities include hypospadias with, often, a bifid scrotum. Intellectual development is usually normal. The main problem faced by these children is recurrent pulmonary aspiration and this is likely to be fatal in infancy if untreated. Urgent prophylactic jejunostomy and, possibly, cervical oesophagostomy are indicated. The oropharyngeal and respiratory problems do improve with time and these patients should be capable of a near normal life span.

The principal anaesthetic problem is one of preventing tracheal aspiration. A technique which has been safely employed includes atropine premedication, passing a nasogastric tube, gaseous induction of anaesthesia with cricoid pressure and intubation under direct vision following suxamethonium [1]. The immature larynx may necessitate the use of a tracheal tube smaller than expected. There are no other reports of anaesthesia in this condition.

Reference

1 Bolsin SN, Gillbe C. *Anaesthesia*, 1985; **40**: 1189–1193.

Osteitis deformans

Paget's disease of bone

Major problem
Pathological fractures

This metabolic disorder is characterised by extensive resorption and replacement of bone. The patients are usually in late middle age or older and of either sex. The bones most frequently affected are skull, pelvis, tibia, femur, humerus, and vertebrae, although any bone may be involved. Bone pain is a common symptom and pathological fractures occur. Collapse of vertebrae may result in spinal cord compression and a marked kyphosis. Atlanto-axial instability is an occasional finding. Increased vascularity develops in the affected areas of bone, eventually leading to the appearance of direct arteriovenous shunts. Cardiac output rises in compensation and high output cardiac failure may be the end result. The serum calcium and phosphate levels are normal, although the alkaline phosphatase is grossly elevated. These patients may be on treatment with steroids, calcitonin or high-dose aspirin.

There are no particular anaesthetic drugs or techniques which are either recommended or contra-indicated for these patients. If they have a kyphosis pulmonary function tests should be performed pre-operatively. The cardiovascular system has to be examined for evidence of heart failure. It is also wise to assess the stability of the neck. Care must be taken with the handling of these patients due to the increased risk of pathological fractures. Vertebral involvement may make the insertion of a spinal or epidural difficult and if there is established spinal cord compression, autonomic hyperreflexia (page 29) may be a problem. If the patient is receiving treatment with steroids, additional cover should be considered, and if the patient is taking aspirin, platelet function tests should be performed.

Further reading

Krane SM. *Clin. Orthoped.* 1977; **127**: 24–31

Osteogenesis imperfecta

Fragilatans ossium

Major problems
Extremely brittle bones
Difficult intubation
Likely association with malignant hyperpyrexia

This rare connective tissue disorder is inherited in an autosomal dominant manner. Two subtypes exist: osteogenesis imperfecta congenita and osteogenesis imperfecta tarda. Babies suffering from the congenita type are born with multiple fractures and do not usually survive beyond childhood. The other type, osteogenesis imperfecta tarda, develops during childhood and may not greatly alter the patient's normal lifespan. There is a defect of collagen formation which results in greatly increased fragility of bones. In addition, these patients have lax ligaments, short stature, kyphoscoliosis, blue sclerae, brittle teeth and slowly progressive deafness. Other associations include inguinal hernia, increased bleeding tendency, congenital heart lesions, cleft palate, spina bifida and metabolic disorders, in particular increased metabolic rate and hyperthermia.

It is clear that handling, positioning and moving these patients must be done with extreme care because of the high risk of fractured limbs. The bones may be so brittle that a fractured humerus may follow application of a blood pressure cuff [1]. Airway and intubation difficulties are also common because pressure from facemask and laryngoscope may fracture the mandible. The teeth are very brittle, mouth opening may be reduced and cervical spine movements may be limited. Intubation should be avoided or approached with great care. Intermittent ketamine has been used successfully. An association has been reported with malignant hyperpyrexia [2]. It is wise therefore to take a careful personal and family history. Avoid the most common malignant hyperpyrexia triggering agents (see page 141) and monitor the patient's temperature throughout anaesthesia. Regional anaesthesia is not contra-indicated and the successful use of an epidural blockade for caesarean section has been reported [3]. The presence of kyphoscoliosis, bleeding tendency and abnormalities of the lumbar spine must however be borne in mind. The possibility of the presence of other congenital disorders, e.g. heart lesions, must be borne in mind during the pre-operative assessment and appropriate management included.

References

1 Oliviero RM. *Anesth. Analg.*, 1973; **52:** 232–236.
2 Rampton AJ, Kelly DA, Shanahan EC, Ingram GS. *Br. J. Anaesth.*, 1984; **56:** 1443–1446.
3 Cunningham AJ, Donnelly M, Comerford J. *Anesthesiology*, 1984; **61:** 91–93.

Osteopetrosis

Marble bone disease, Albers-Schonberg disease,
recessive osteopetrosis, dominant osteopetrosis

Major problems
Brittle bones
Anaemia

There are two varieties of osteopetrosis: a mild form being inherited in an autosomal dominant fashion and a more severe form which is autosomal recessive in nature. Both types are characterised by abnormally dense sclerotic patches of bone. In the benign dominant form many patients are asymptomatic and the disorder may be diagnosed as an incidental finding on routine X-ray. The generalised sclerosis of bone leads to a reduction in the size of the medullary cavity and bone pain is often a feature. The bones of the skull may be thickened leading to frontal bossing and the possibility of cranial nerve palsies, especially of cranial nerves 2, 3 and 7. These patients usually have a normal life span. In the more severe recessive form there is often a complete obliteration of the marrow cavity leading to severe anaemia. Hepatosplenomegaly is also present and these patients die in infancy.

In view of the increased brittleness of the bones care should be taken in moving and positioning these patients. Anaemia may result from the marrow sclerosis and the blood count should be checked. If hepatosplenomegaly is present it is wise to check liver function. There are no particular drugs or techniques which are contra-indicated.

Further reading

Beighton P, Horan F, Mamersma H. *Postgrad. Med. J.* 1977; **53:** 507–521.

Pacemakers

Major problems
Diathermy interference
Dislodged pacing wire

Pacemakers are inserted for a number of conditions and it is important to know the nature of the underlying condition which necessitates the presence of the pacemaker. There may be significant additional cardiovascular disease. If the pacemaker is a permanently implanted type its function should be checked pre-operatively. If the pacemaker is a temporary external type it is important to ensure that the controls are readily accessible at all times. Antibiotic prophylaxis against bacterial endocarditis should be considered.

There is no constraint to the anaesthetic technique except that due to the underlying cardiac pathology. The ECG must be continually monitored throughout the procedure. Modern pacemakers should not be affected by diathermy but it is a wise precaution to avoid diathemy and all radar and radiotelemetry devices if possible. If diathermy is required the indifferent plate and diathermy machine should be positioned as far away from the pacemaker as possible. Most pacemakers may be converted from the synchronous (demand) mode into the asynchronous (fixed rate) mode by application of an external magnet. Such a magnet should be available in the anaesthetic room. Avoid trauma to the area of the pacemaker. If central venous cannulation is necessary it must be done with great care so as not to dislodge the pacing wires. Disturbances in blood gases and electrolytes must be avoided if possible because these may change the capturing threshold of the pacemaker system.

Further reading

Zaidan JR. *Anesthesiology*, 1984; **60:** 319–334.

Paramyotonia congenita

Eulenberg's disease

Major problem

Myotonia (mild) exacerbated by coldness

This autosomal dominant condition is characterised by weakness and myotonia on exposure to cold. The weakness is not improved by exercise and responds to quinidine therapy. There is otherwise a strong similarity to myotonia congenita.

Anaesthesia does not present a great problem in this condition. Hypothermia should be avoided because this exacerbates the myotonia. The patient's temperature should be continuously monitored, a warm water circulating mattress placed on the operating table and covers kept on all parts of the patient which do not have to be uncovered. Suxamethonium should be avoided in all myotonias.

Further reading

Cobham IG, Davis HS. *Anesth. Analg.*, 1964, **43:** 22−29.
Ellis FR. *Br. J. Anaesth.*, 1980; **52:** 153−164.
Ellis FR. *Br. J. Anaesth.*, 1974; **46:** 603−612.

Paraplegia

Spinal cord transection

Major problems
Autonomic hyperreflexia
Avoid suxamethonium

Complete section of the spinal cord produces loss of motor function and sensation below the site of the lesion. Reflex responses may still be present. If the lesion is above the mid-thoracic level vascular instability may result, in particular noxious stimulation below the level of the lesion may produce an exaggerated hypertensive response associated with bradycardia, sweating, flushing and piloerection (autonomic hyperreflexia). In addition, the higher the lesion, the greater will be the respiratory embarrassment as more of the lower intercostal muscles are paralysed.

In the pre-operative assessment of these patients the level of damage to the spinal cord should be noted. If autonomic hyperreflexia is likely then see page 29. If the thoracic level is involved the patient's respiratory reserve should be assessed. Problems with coughing and clearing secretions may be encountered in the postoperative period and physiotherapy is important to lessen the likelihood of chest infection. Suxamethonium is safe only for the first 7–10 days. After that it should not be used because an exaggerated hyperkalaemic response may ensue. Nondepolarising muscle relaxants present no problems. In the acute stages the spine may be unstable and so moving and positioning of the patient should be done with care. In the later stages positioning may again be a problem due to contractures and pressure sores. The patient's temperature regulation is usually impaired and so exposed areas of skin should be covered and the body temperature monitored throughout. As time progresses renal function often deteriorates and it is wise to assess renal function pre-operatively.

Further reading

Tobey RE. *Anesthesiology*, 1970; **32:** 359–364.
Hassan HG. *Anaesthesia*, 1974; **29:** 629–630.

Parkinson's disease

Paralysis agitans

Major problem
Potential cardiovascular instability

Parkinson's disease is a disorder of the basal ganglia usually affecting the older age groups, particularly the over 60s. It is characterised by weakness, rigidity and tremor. There is a paucity of movement, mask-like facies, and sometimes dysarthria and increased salivation.

These patients do not present any major problems for anaesthesia. They are usually on therapy with L-dopa, which should be stopped 12—24 hours pre-operatively. Hypotension, or occasionally hypertension, is likely if L-dopa is continued, although it has been reported in patients in whom the L-dopa was stopped 24 hours pre-operatively.

Theoretically, phenothiazines and butyrophenones (e.g. droperidol, haloperidol, chorpromazine) are contra-indicated and they should therefore be avoided, although they have been given to Parkinsonian patients without problems. The patient may be receiving additional drug therapy with antidepressants and anticholinergics. If an anti-emetic is required, cyclizine is the drug of choice.

Further reading

Azar I. *Anesthesiology*, 1984, **61:** 173—187
Gravlee GP. *Anesth. Analg.*, 1980; **59:** 444—446.
Ngai SH. *Anesthesiology*, 1972, **37:** 344—351.

Paroxysmal nocturnal haemoglobinuria

Major problems
Venous thrombosis
Bleeding tendency
Anaemia

This is a rare chronic haemolytic anaemia in which the cell membranes have an abnormal sensitivity to lysis by complement. Symptoms may be the result of a bleeding tendency or venous thrombosis. The former is due to thrombocytopaenia and the latter due to abnormal platelet function. Renal or hepatic vein thrombosis (Budd-Chiari syndrome) are common complications.

Transfusion, if necessary, should be with washed red cells as foreign plasma may activate complement and lead to further haemolysis of the patient's erythrocytes. The removal of leucocytes also reduces the risk of leucocytic sensitisation. Pre-operative exchange transfusion may be necessary to reduce the proportion of abnormal cells. Subcutaneous heparin, together with adequate hydration, may reduce the likelihood of venous thrombosis which is most common in the postoperative period — complement levels are at their peak at about the fourth day.

Intravenous agents are prone to complement activation and should be avoided — an inhalational induction of anaesthesia or a regional local anaesthetic technique should be seriously considered. Avoid any agents with a reputation for anaphylactoid reaction. Nitrous oxide is known to cause megaloblastic bone marrow changes and thus it would seem sensible to avoid it in an already anaemic patient with a hypoplastic marrow. Infection causes complement activation and thus prophylactic gut decontamination and specific antibiotic therapy where necessary should be started.

Further reading

Taylor MB, Whitwam JG, Worsley A. *Anaesthesia*, 1987; **42**: 639.

Pemphigus and pemphigoid

Major problems
Minor local trauma results in bulla formation
Avoid airway manipulations and intubation if
   possible

These two skin conditions differ somewhat in their aetiology, treatment and prognosis. They are, however, being considered together here because they are conditions of similar superficial appearance and they share a number of common anaesthetic problems.

Both are characterised by the appearance of large tense bullae in the skin or mucous membranes, in particular following a minor episode of local trauma. Pemphigus and bullous pemphigoid lesions usually spontaneously resolve without scarring. In cicatricial pemphigoid, however, scarring develops in the site of the bullae which may lead to contracture formation. When this is close to the site of a body aperture then stenosis of this aperture results. Scarring and cicatrix formation is a particular problem when it affects the larynx or trachea. The patient may be malnourished due to the presence of frequent intra-oral lesions and lesions in the larynx may produce hoarseness and stridor.

An association has been suggested between pemphigoid and myasthenia gravis, systemic lupus erythematosis, rheumatoid arthritis, pernicious anaemia and primary liver cirrhosis.

The most important consideration in these patients is to avoid all forms of trauma to skin or mucous membrane, however minor it may seem to be. The patient should be lifted and moved very carefully. It is wise to avoid all airway manipulations if possible, including oral or nasal airways, tracheal tubes and face-masks. If these are necessary, use plenty of lubricant and be VERY GENTLE. Trauma to the mucous membranes may produce bulla formation which can obstruct the airway. If the patient has had previous airway manipulations or if there is a history of stridor or dyspnoea then laryngeal or tracheal stenosis should be suspected. The patient is likely to be receiving steroid therapy and so peri-operative cover will be needed. A technique using intermittent intravenous diazepam and ketamine has been successfully used in these patients.

Electrolyte disturbances and hypo-albuminaemia occur and these should be assessed pre-operatively.

Further reading

Drenger B, Zidenbaum M, Reifen E, Leitersdorf E. *Anaesthesia*, 1986, **41**: 1029−1031.
Vatashsky E, Aronson HB. *Anaesthesia*, 1982, **37**: 1195−1197.

Peroneal muscular atrophy

Charcot-Marie-Tooth disease

Major problem
Possible diminished respiratory reserve

This rare syndrome of peripheral nerve degeneration is inherited in an autosomal dominant fashion. Demyelination of peripheral axons results in weakness in the limbs, especially the legs and feet. Exacerbation of the disease by pregnancy has been reported, with weakness extending to the proximal muscles and reducing respiratory reserve. These severe symptoms resolved once the pregnancy had ended. Myocardial involvement has been reported, in particular conduction abnormalities.

If the patient is only minimally affected then anaesthesia should not present any problems. It will be necessary to assess cardio-respiratory reserve before anaesthesia in patients who are more severely affected. These patients may also require postoperative ventilatory support. Suxamethonium has been used without problem, although it may be theoretically contra-indicated if there is a large amount of denervated muscle. There is no evidence to suggest that the condition is made worse by anaesthesia.

Further reading

Brian JE, Boyles GD, Quirk JG, Clark RB. *Anesthesiology*, 1987, **66**: 410−412.

Phaeochromocytoma

Major problems
Cardiovascular instability
Sudden episodes of hypertension
Sudden episodes of serious cardiac arrhythmias

A phaeochromocytoma is a tumour (usually benign) which secretes adrenaline and noradrenaline into the circulation. Clinical presentation is classically with paroxysmal hypertension, but sustained hypertension, headache, palpitations, sweating, dyspnoea and abdominal pains are also described. Phaeochromocytomas may form part of the multiple endocrine adenomatosis syndromes (see page 22). Diagnosis is usually made by detecting raised serum catecholamine levels and raised urinary excretion of catecholamine metabolites.

Anaesthesia in the presence of untreated phaeochromocytoma is hazardous and carries a high mortality, although if previously diagnosed and carefully managed this high mortality can be eliminated. The cornerstone of successful management in these patients is careful pre-operative assessment. The patients have a chronically contracted plasma volume. Alpha adrenergic blockade should be begun several days pre-operatively and surgery postponed until the blood pressure is stable. Phenoxybenzamine is the usual drug of choice. Other drugs with alpha blocking action have been used, however, including prazosin and chlorpromazine, and it may be necessary to include treatment with a beta blocker (e.g. propranolol) in addition to the alpha blocker. Labetalol has been used but is less effective than the other drugs. An adequate premedication is advisable to reduce anxiety. Most general anaesthetic agents and techniques have been used with success. The following drugs do have theoretical contraindications: tubocurarine and morphine may release histamine which stimulates catecholamine release from the tumour; halothane and cyclopropane may increase the incidence of arrhythmias; gallamine causes a tachycardia; suxamethonium fasiculations may mechanically stimulate the tumour. It is wise, therefore, to avoid these agents. It is essential to maintain a good depth of anaesthesia in order to blunt the hypertensive episodes. These episodes are not uncommon with handling of the tumour and are best treated with phentolamine IV. Sodium nitroprusside and intravenous nitrate have also been used to good effect.

Following removal of the tumour, hypotension is common and usually responds to the rapid intravenous administration of fluid. Vasopressors are occasionally required, e.g. phenylephrine or noradrenaline, and it is wise to have them to hand. The high levels of catecholamines often produce serious cardiac arrhythmias which may be managed with lignocaine or propranolol IV. An indwelling arterial line and a central venous pressure line are recommended in addition to the usual routine monitoring. Reports have demonstrated discrepancies between left and right heart filling pressures in these patients and a good argument can be advanced for the pre-operative insertion of a pulmonary flotation catheter. Cardiovascular instability often continues into the postoperative period and monitoring should therefore continue as long as necessary on a high dependency unit.

There are numerous case reports of the anaesthetic management of phaeochromocytoma in the literature. The majority of these appear in the references section of the two reviews cited.

Further reading

Desmonts JM, Marty J. *Br. J. Anaesth.*, 1984; **56**: 781–789.
Pratilas V, Pratila MG. *Can. Anaesth. Soc. J.*, 1979; **26**: 253–259.

Pharyngeal teratoma

Major problem
Airway obstruction

This rare congenital lesion presents at birth with a bulky tumour protruding through the mouth. The tumour bulk may be such as to distort the face and mouth and cause airway obstruction. Treatment is by surgical excision.

The main consideration in these patients is that of maintaining the airway. Facial distortion may prevent any use of a face-mask. The child may need immediate tracheal intubation or tracheostomy at birth. Manipulations in the airway of these patients should be performed with great care because the tumor is usually very vascular and may be quite friable.

Further reading

Diaz JH, Stedman PM, LeTard FX. *Anesthesiology,* 1984; **61:** 608−610.

Phenylketonuria

Major problem
Possible hypoglycaemia

This autosomal recessive conditon is characterised by an absence of the enzyme phenylalanine hydroxylase. This leads to an increase in phenylalanine concentration in blood and of phenylalanine excretion in the urine. These patients have defective pigmentation and a defect in CNS myelin formation. Unless prescribed a low phenylalanine diet soon after birth they become mentally retarded. They also frequently suffer from fits.

Premedication may be unpredictable and pre-operative management of these patients may be a problem if they are mentally retarded. An increased sensitivity to opiates, barbiturates and other CNS depressants has been reported. No difficulties have been reported however with the use of volatile anaesthetic agents. There is an increased susceptibility to hypoglycaemia and so prolonged pre-operative starvation should be avoided or glucose supplied by intravenous infusion. If the patient is on treatment for fits this must be continued throughout the perioperative period and anaesthetic agents known to exacerbate this condition (e.g. enflurane, methohexitone) be avoided. These patients have sensitive skins which can be easily traumatised by adhesive plaster.

Further reading

Jackson SH. In: *Anaesthesia and Uncommon Diseases: pathophysiologic and clinical correlations*, 2nd edn, 1981. Ed. Katz J, Benumof J, Kadis LB. WB Saunders, Philadelphia, pp. 35−40.

Pneumatosis cystoides intestinalis

Major problem
Cyst expansion with nitrous oxide

In this condition, gas filled cysts form in the walls of the intestine. They are often asymptomatic but may give rise to symptoms of diarrhoea, abdominal pain, excessive flatus and bleeding. Treatment is the inhalation of a high concentration of oxygen.

The only anaesthetic consideration in this condition is the avoidance of nitrous oxide. Nitrous oxide diffuses into the cysts causing expansion and possible rupture. The patient should therefore receive 100% oxygen, or oxygen enriched air, during the course of anaesthesia.

Further reading

Sutton DN, Poskitt KR. *Anaesthesia*, 1984; **39**: 776−779.

Polyarteritis nodosa

Periarteritis nodosa

Major problems
Possible myocardial ischaemia
Sensitivity to vaso-active drugs

This condition is characterised by a widespread vasculitis which leads to weakening and dilatation of the walls of arteries. Thrombosis and aneurysms develop in many small arteries and the exact clinical presentation depends upon the sites of the lesions. Renal failure may result from vasculitis in the renal bed and pulmonary fibrosis from lesions in the lungs. The coronary vessels may also be involved, leading to myocardial ischaemia. The disease undergoes a relapsing and remitting course.

Pre-operative assessment should include tests of pulmonary function and enquiries regarding myocardial ischaemic symptoms. The patients are often taking steroids and appropriate steroid cover should be considered. If ischaemic heart disease is present care must be taken to maintain the normal myocardial oxygen supply/demand ratio. The patients are often hypertensive and may exhibit an unusual sensitivity to vasopressor and vaso-depressor agents. Arthritis in the temporomandibular joints or crico-arytenoid joints may occasionally give rise to airway or intubation difficulties. Acute pharyngeal oedema has been reported in this disease [1].

Reference

1 Martin TH. *Can. Med. Assoc. J.*, 1969; **101**: 229–231.

Further reading

Bellamy N, Kean WF, Buchanan WW. *Hospital Update*, 1984; **10**: 135–146.

Porphyria

Major problem
Acute attack precipitated
by many anaesthetic agents

The porphyrias comprise a family of hereditary metabolic disorders of porphyrin metabolism. They are generally classified into two major groups, designated acute and non-acute or hepatic and non-hepatic. These two groupings are not identical. It is the acute group which is of importance to anaesthetists and includes acute intermittent porphyria, variegate porphyria and hereditary coproporphyria. Acute attacks of porphyria may be precipitated by a number of situations, including pregnancy, infection and a number of drugs. An acute attack results in severe symptoms and can be fatal. Symptoms include acute abdominal pain and vomiting, paralyses, sensory disturbances, psychiatric or psychological disorders, fits, visual disturbances, hypertension and tachycardia.

The most important consideration for the anaesthetist is the avoidance of all precipitating factors. The possibility of porphyria must always be borne in mind with the association of an acute abdomen and other unexpected symptoms or signs. The list of drugs which must be avoided is considerable and for a full list the reader is referred to a standard medical text [1]. Those of most relevance to anaesthesia, which must be *avoided* include: thiopentone and all barbiturates, all benzodiazepines, ethyl alcohol, alcuronium, amitriptyline, chlormethiazole, chlorpropamide, cimetidine, clonidine, cocaine, ergot preparations, erythromycin, hydralazine, methyldopa, metoclopramide, metronidazole, nikethamide, pentazocine, phenoxybenzamine, phenytoin, phenylbutazone, piritramide, spironolactone, steroids, sulphonamides, theophylline, tolbutamide.

This second list includes a number of drugs which *appear to be safe*, although evidence is conflicting for some which are marked with an asterisk. Ketamine, etomidate*, propofol*, nitrous oxide, opiates, buprenorphine, atropine, hyoscine, diethylether, suxamethonium, tubocurarine, pancuronium*, gallamine, enflurane*, halothane*, isoflurane, chlorpromazine, promazine, promethazine, chloral hydrate, paraldehyde, pentolinium, propranolol, procaine, cyclopropane, neostigmine, disopyramide, droperidol, heparin, labetalol, oxytocin, paracetamol, phentolamine.

There is no specific contra-indication to local and regional anaesthesia in these patients but in view of the natural course of the disease, including sensory and motor disturbances, many people feel it wise to avoid these techniques. Bupivacaine has been reported to be safe but lignocaine may not be.

Reference

1 Goldberg A, Moore MR, McColl KEL, Brodie MJ. In: *Oxford Textbook of Medicine*, 2nd edn, 1987, Ed. Weatherall DJ, Ledingham JGG, Warrell DA. Oxford Medical Publications, chapter 9, pp. 136–145.

Further reading

Murphy PC. *Br. J. Anaesth.*, 1964; **36:** 801–812.
Mustajoki P, Heinonen J. *Anesthesiology,* 1980; **53:** 15–20.

Prader Willi syndrome

Prader Labhart Willi syndrome

Major problems
Obesity
Tendency to hypoglycaemia

The combination of neonatal hypotonia, mental deficiency, hyperphagia, obesity, dental caries, hypogonadism, and cryptorchidism makes up the Prader Willi syndrome. As an infant the patient is hypotonic and apathetic but as childhood advances, uncontrollable eating begins and the child rapidly becomes grossly obese. Diabetes mellitus commonly develops at about ten years of age.

These patients may develop hypoglycaemia if fasted for more than a few hours and therefore frequent estimates of blood sugar, together with an intravenous glucose infusion are recommended. There are no specific anaesthetic agents or techniques which are either recommended or contra-indicated. The response to muscle relaxants is normal. The gross obesity may be a problem during aneaesthesia and in the postoperative period (see page 178). Some patients may have developed a Pickwickian-type syndrome with hypoventilation and cor pulmonale and such patients are a high risk for anaesthesia (see page 20). A period of postoperative controlled ventilation may be necessary. The generalised weakness reduces the effectiveness of the cough reflex resulting in repeated episodes of tracheal aspiration. Disturbances of temperature regulation have been described [1] and it is wise to monitor the patient's temperature continuously throughout anaesthesia. Unexpected cardiac arrhythmias have also been reported [2].

References

1 Mayhew JF, Taylor B. *Can. Anaesth. Soc. J.*, 1983; **30:** 565−566.
2 Milliken RA, Weintraub DM. *Anesthesiology*, 1975; **43:** 590−592.

Further reading

Palmer SK, Atlee JL. *Anesthesiology*, 1975; **44:** 161–163.
Yamashita M, Koishi K, Yamaya R, Tsubo T, Matsuki A, Oyama T. *Can. Anaesth. Soc. J.,* 1983; **30:** 179–184.

Prinzmetal's variant angina

Major problem
Potential myocardial ischaemia

The pathophysiology of this condition is thought to be spasm of a coronary artery. If the artery is already partially occluded by atheroma then a critical reduction in blood supply results. However, it has also been shown to occur, by angiography, in patients with normal coronary arteries. Classically chest pain is not precipitated by exercise. In the case report cited [1] pain appeared coincidental with a reduction in blood pressure as an extradural block was being established. The classic ECG changes consist of a raised ST segment over the affected area with a depressed ST segment in the opposite leads. The symptoms and spasm are relieved promptly by glyceryl trinitrate.

Calcium antagonists are also a useful treatment and the patient may already be taking one. They must not be stopped pre-operatively. Propranolol may exacerbate the condition and should be avoided. There are otherwise no specific recommendations or contra-indications for anaesthesia.

Reference

1 Krantz EM, Viljeon JF, Gilbert MS. *Br. J. Anaesth.*, 1980; **52**: 945.

Progeria

Hutchinson-Gilford syndrome

Major problems
Myocardial ischaemia
Intubation difficulties

This rare autosomal recessive condition is characterised by premature aging. The child may appear normal at birth but the accelerated aging process begins at about 6−12 months and the patients do not usually survive beyond 20 years of age. There is a rapidly progressive development of ischaemic heart disease, hypertension, cerebrovascular disease and arthritis. Intellectual development is usually normal. They have thin skin, alopecia, brittle bones and a thin malnourished appearance. Mandibular hypoplasia with micrognathia has been reported.

Anaesthetic management of these patients is principally the same as for adults of advanced years suffering the normal aging process. The patient should be managed as though they have significant ischaemic heart disease. Positioning and moving the patient must be undertaken with care in view of their brittle bones and thin skin. The presence of mandibular hypoplasia may make airway management and intubation difficult. Furthermore, the patient is likely to have a poorly developed larynx and a tracheal tube of a size smaller than expected may be required.

Further reading

Chapin JW, Kahne J. *Anesth. Analg.*, 1979; **58**: 424−425.

Prolonged QT syndrome

Long QT syndrome, Jervell-Lange-Nielson syndrome,
cardioauditory syndrome, Romano-Ward syndrome

Major problem
Serious cardiac arrhythmias

Prolongation of the QT interval on the ECG may be either congenital or acquired. The congenital form may be associated with
nerve deafness when it forms the Jervell-Lange-Nielson syndrome (cardioauditory syndrome). Acquired prolongation of the
QT interval may be secondary to myocarditis, myocardial infarction, hypokalaemia, hypocalcaemia or drug ingestion. The significance of the prolonged QT interval is that there may be
unexpected episodes of ventricular dysrhythmias which result in
palpitations, syncope or even sudden death. These episodes may
be precipitated by strenuous activity or stress, including surgery
and anaesthesia. The normal QT interval varies with the heart
rate and is approximately 0.42 seconds at a heart rate of 50 per
minute, falling to 0.30 seconds at a heart rate of 100 per minute.
It is an imbalance of the right and left cardiac sympathetic supply
which is the presumed pathology, overactivity of the left side
resulting in the prolonged QT interval. Local block or surgical
ablation of the left stellate ganglion has been reported to effect a
cure.

The principal consideration of anaesthesia in these patients is
the prevention of dysrhythmias. Both physical and psychological
stress may accentuate the problem and should be avoided. Gentle
intubation is advisable, with possibly the use of topical local
anaesthesia. The presence of a tube in the trachea may stimulate
dysrhythmias and it is therefore wise to extubate the patient
whilst still anaesthetised. Propranolol has been shown to reduce
the risk and this should be started pre-operatively and be available intra-operatively. A good dose of a sedative premedicant is
helpful. Continuous ECG monitoring is essential throughout.
Drugs which have been *safely* used include: thiopentone, suxamethonium, nitrous oxide, enflurane, isoflurane, fentanyl,

211

morphine, hyoscine, alcuronium and vecuronium. The following drugs have been associated with problems and are best *avoided:* halothane, gallamine, pancuronium, atropine, quinidine, procainamide and ketamine. The dysrhythmias have been treated with lignocaine, digoxin and phenytoin but these drugs do not always work.

Further reading

Blair JR, Pruett JK, Crumrine RS, Balser JS. *Anesthesiology*, 1987; **67:** 442–443.

Brown M, Liberthson RR, Ali HH, Lowenstein E. *Anesthesiology*, 1981; **55:** 586–589.

Carlock FJ, Brown M, Brown EM. *Can. Anaesth. Soc. J.*, 1984; **31:** 83–85.

Freshwater JV. *Br. J. Anaesth.*, 1984; **56:** 655–657.

Medak R, Benumof JL. *Br. J. Anaesth.*, 1983; **55:** 361–364.

O'Callaghan AC, Normandale JP, Morgan M. *Anaesth. Intensive Care*, 1982; **10:** 50–55.

Wig J, Bali IM, Singh RG, Kataria RN, Khattri HN. *Anaesthesia*, 1979; **34:** 37–40.

Wilton NCT, Hantler CB. *Anesth. Analg.*, 1987; **66:** 357–360.

Protein C deficiency

Major problem
Venous thrombosis

Protein C is an essential circulating anticoagulant factor derived from vitamin K. Deficiency of this protein may be acquired in liver disease, disseminated intravascular coagulation, the adult respiratory distress syndrome, the postoperative period, or inherited as an autosomal dominant trait. There is an increase in blood coagulability with an increase in tendency to thrombosis and thrombophlebitis. Fresh frozen plasma is rich in protein C and may be used for replacement therapy. The patient may also be receiving heparin or other anticoagulant therapy.

Anaesthetic procedures should be designed to minimise any venous thrombosis. Prophylaxis against deep vein thrombosis must be considered. Thrombosis may occur in any vein in the body, including superficial veins, resulting in patches of necrosis over pressure points. The pressure on the inside of the trachea from an overinflated cuff may also result in thrombosis and oedema of the tracheal mucosa with subsequent stenosis.

Further reading

Wetzel RC, Marsh BR, Yater M, Casella JF. *Anesth. Analg.*, 1986; **65**: 982−984.

Prune belly syndrome

Abdominal muscular deficiency syndrome

Major problems
Postoperative respiratory insufficiency
Associated renal failure

This congenital disorder is characterised by agenesis of the anterior abdominal wall musculature. The majority of these patients have additional congenital abnormalities, the urinary tract is commonly involved. Many have small dysplastic kidneys and renal failure, heart lesions and pulmonary hypoplasia have also been reported.

The patient's respiratory system must be carefully assessed pre-operatively and any existing infection brought under control before considering anaesthesia. The possibility of other congenital disorders must be borne in mind. The urea and electrolytes should be measured. Drugs which rely solely on the kidneys for excretion should be avoided. There are otherwise no particular anaesthetic agents or techniques which are contra-indicated. There is no good evidence to suggest that muscle relaxants should be avoided. An anaesthetic technique employing controlled ventilation is recommended. The principal problem which will be faced is one of postoperative respiratory insufficiency. The patients are unable to cough very well so regular physiotherapy will be necessary.

A period of postoperative ventilatory support may also be required. The potent analgesics which are also respiratory depressants and cough suppressants are not contra-indicated but should be given with care. The weak cough reflex may also lead to an increased incidence of pulmonary aspiration of gastric contents. Special care must therefore be taken in those patients who are more prone to the regurgitation of gastric contents.

Further reading

Hannington-Kiff JG. *Br. J. Anaesth*, 170; **42:** 649−652.
Henderson AM, Vallis CJ, Sumner E. *Anaesthesia*, 1987; **42:** 54−60.
Karamanian A, Kravath R, Nagashima H, Gentsh HH. *Br. J. Anaesth*, 1974; **46:** 897−899.

Pseudoxanthoma elasticum

Groenblad-Strandberg syndrome

Major problems
Fragile skin
Fragile blood vessels
Avoid hypertension

This genetically determined disorder of elastic tissue formation is inherited recessively and is of widely varying severity. Lifespan is not affected. Changes are most obvious in the skin, although defects in the walls of blood vessels are the most important. The eye (retinal haemorrhages), the gastro-intestinal system (bleeding), the cardiovascular system (hypertension, angina, coronary artery disease, myocardial infarction) and the brain and cerebrovascular system (intracranial haemorrhage, psychiatric disturbance) are commonly affected.

The cardiovascular manifestations are probably the most important to anaesthesia [1]. A technique appropriate to patients with coronary artery disease is recommended. The blood pressure should be monitored carefully and hypertension avoided in view of the weakness in many arteries. It is best to avoid using an indwelling arterial cannula. Intravenous infusions are difficult to maintain *in situ* and regularly become displaced. The thin friable skin and mucous membranes are easily traumatised and care must be taken with all handling and instrumentation of the patient. Even the insertion of a nasogastric tube must be viewed with caution lest bleeding of the nose, pharynx or gastro-intestinal tract occurs. In one case report [2] rigidity and deformity of the larynx was noted, making tracheal intubation difficult.

References

1 Wilson Krechel SL, Ramirez-Inawat RC, Fabian LW. *Anesth. Analg.*, 1981; **60:** 344–347.
2 Levitt MWD, Collison JM. *Anaesth. Intensive Care*, 1982; **10:** 62–64.

Pulmonary fibrosis
(secondary to antineoplastics)

Major problem
Pulmonary oxygen toxicity

Many of the antineoplastic agents can cause pulmonary toxicity. This does not occur in every patient and may range from minimal pulmonary infiltration to massive fatal fibrosis. The toxicity appears to be made worse by a high inspired oxygen concentration and has a clinical appearance resembling the adult respiratory distress syndrome. It must be remembered that the association between oxygen toxicity and certain antineoplastics is not proven beyond all doubt. Bleomycin appears to be the most potent agent with respect to this problem, but the following antineoplastics may also be implicated [1]: mitomycin, doxarubicin, daunorubicin, dactinomycin, carmustine, cytarabine, methotrexate, procarbazine, cyclophosphamide, busulphan, chlorambucil, melphalan.

The most common recommendation is to use an $F_{I}O_2$ of 0.25 throughout. In view of the risk of hypoxaemia oxygenation should be continously monitored. A pulse oximeter [3] or intravascular P_{O_2} electrode [4] have both been recommended. Postoperative oxygen therapy should also be limited and it may be wise to monitor fluid balance with extra care. One report examined a series of patients in whom the mean $F_{I}O_2$ was 0.41. No pulmonary problems were reported, which suggests that oxygen may not be the only factor involved [5].

References

1 Klein DS, Wilds PR. *Can. Anaesth. Soc. J.,* 1983; **30** 399−405.
2 Douglas MJ, Coppin CML. *Can. Anaesth. Soc. J.,* 1980; **27:** 449−454.
3 Brodsky JB, Shulman MS. *Can. Anaesth. Soc. J.,* 1984; **31:** 488−489.
4 Oxorn DC, Chung DC, Lam AM. *Can. Anaesth. Soc. J.,* 1984; **31:** 200−205.
5 LaMantia KR, Glick JH, Marshall BE. *Anesthesiology,* 1984; **60:** 65−67.

Pyruvate dehydrogenase deficiency

Lactic acidosis

Major problem
Chronic lactic acidosis

This inborn error of metabolism (enzyme deficiency) results in an inability to convert pyruvate into acetyl CoA for normal metabolic processes. The result is an abnormal accumulation of lactate and pyruvate. The patients have a chronic metabolic acidosis with markedly raised serum lactate concentration. The patients usually have a degree of neurological dysfuntion and may be lethargic and irritable. Stress may exacerbate the neurological symptoms. This defect is unlikely to be compatible with survival beyond childhood.

Pre-operative assessment of these patients must include full assessment of their acid base status and lactate levels. Any other predisposing factors for acidosis, e.g. sepsis or hypothermia, should be sought and corrected. Anaesthetic techniques using thiopentone for induction of anaesthesia and maintenance with isoflurane or a neurolept combination of agents have both been safely used. Lactate-containing intravenous fluids must be avoided. Frequent intravenous boluses of bicarbonate will be necessary to prevent excessive acidosis. Children with primary lactic acidosis are prone to central respiratory depression and so careful observation for hypoventilation is required in the postoperative period.

Further reading

Dierdorf SF, McNeice WL. *Can. Anaesth. Soc. J.*, 1983; **30**: 413–416.

Reye's syndrome

Major problems
Liver failure
Raised intracranial pressure

This disease, of unknown aetiology, usually follows an acute viral illness in children. A possible association with aspirin ingestion has recently led to the withdrawal of aspirin-containing medicines for children. A severe encephalopathy develops together with fatty degeneration of the viscera, particularly the liver. There is an increase in blood ammonia and transaminase levels, together with other stigmata of liver disease, e.g. coagulopathy. If left untreated the mortality is high (22−54%), uncontrollable intracranial hypertension usually being the terminal event. A number of treatments have been proposed including blood-free hypothermic total body washout.

Intubation and ventilation are recommended in order to control intracranial pressure. Mannitol, dexamethasone, barbiturate coma and hypothermia may also be used. Any anaesthetic technique which promotes reduction of intracranial pressure is acceptable. Care must be taken with all drugs which are metabolised by the liver. They may need to be given in reduced dosage and their duration of action may be prolonged. It is wise to avoid volatile anaesthetic agents.

Further reading

Talmage EA, Thomas JM, Weeks JH. *Anesth. Analg.*, 1973; **52**: 563−569.

Rheumatoid arthritis

Major problems
Possible intubation difficulties
Atlanto-axial instability
Difficulty in positioning and moving the patient
Fragile veins

Rheumatoid arthritis is a chronic inflammatory disorder, principally affecting the joints. Any joint in the body may be affected to a greater or lesser degree. Rheumatoid nodules may also occur in other organs, in particular the lungs, resulting in pulmonary infiltration and fibrosis. There is an association with amyloidosis (page 13) and the patient may be anaemic.

Problems are many with these patients. Arthritis affecting the temporomandibular joint, arytenoid joints and neck may make intubation difficult. Furthermore, many of these patients have instability of the atlanto-axial joint and it is important to avoid flexion of the head on the neck. They are often on a number of medications, several of which are known to be nephrotoxic. It is wise, therefore, to include a pre-operative assessment of renal function. Peri-operative steroid cover may be needed. There may be considerable deformity of many joints and care should therefore be taken with the positioning of the patient and the protection of pressure points. The patients are often relatively immobile, increasing the risk of deep venous thrombosis. The skin is thin and fragile and venepuncture may be difficult.

Reference

1 Jenkins LC, McGraw RW. *Can. Anaesth. Soc. J.*, 1969; **16**: 407−415.

Rubenstein-Taybi syndrome

Broad thumb-hallux syndrome

Major problems
Tracheal aspiration
Cardiac dysrhythmias

Patients with this syndrome have broad thumbs, broad great toes, facial abnormalities and mental retardation. Congenital heart disease is common and may take the form of any of the large variety of structural or conduction abnormalities. The patients also suffer from repeated episodes of tracheal aspiration resulting in chronic lung disease.

There are two separate reports of anaesthesia for the same patient on different occasions. The main problem encountered was that of cardiac dysrhythmias precipitated on separate occasions by suxamethonium, neostigmine with atropine, and pethidine. It is therefore essential to monitor these patients carefully and to avoid drugs which may induce cardiac irritability. Antibiotic prophylaxis against bacterial endocarditis should be considered if structural heart lesions are present. Difficulties with excessive oropharyngeal secretions were also reported, despite antisialogogue premedication. It would seem to be wise to intubate these patients for every procedure, even those of a minor nature, and not to extubate them until fully awake.

Further reading

Stirt JA. *Anesth. Analg.*, 1981; **60:** 534−536.
Stirt JA. *Anesthesiology*, 1982; **57:** 429.

Sarcoidosis

Major problems
Restrictive lung disease
Multiple system involvement

Sarcoidosis is a chronic granulomatous disease of unknown aetiology. Granulomas may develop in almost any tissue of the body, in particular lung, liver, spleen, skin, eyes, bones and lymph nodes. The condition undergoes spontaneous remission in the majority of patients, although in about 25% it is slowly and relentlessly progressive. Pulmonary infiltration results in a restrictive type of lung disorder with decreased vital capacity and decreased functional residual capacity. Myocardial involvement may produce heart block, heart failure or paroxysmal dysrhythmias. Arthritis, uveitis, impaired liver function, anaemia, thrombocytopaenia and hypercalcaemia are also common.

If the disease does not interfere with daily living then anaesthesia is likely to be uneventful and to pose no problems. If symptoms exist then investigations appropriate to the affected system should be carried out, e.g. pulmonary function tests, full blood count, liver function tests. If lung problems are severe then cor pulmonale may result and invasive cardiac monitoring will be necessary. Hypercalcaemia is a common finding in association with sarcoidosis and it is wise to measure the serum calcium level pre-operatively. Arthritis is present in many patients with sarcoidosis and care with positioning the patient under anaesthesia is important. Arthritis affecting the temporomandibular joint may hinder mouth opening and make for difficulties in intubation. Granulomas may additionally be present in the larynx. In one case descibed [1] a regular sized tracheal tube was a tight fit and postoperative laryngeal oedema led to a stormy postoperative course. The authors recommend a smaller than usual tracheal tube and advise consideration of prophylactic dexamethasone if there is any possibility of laryngeal involvement. The patient may be on steroid therapy and so appropriate extra steroid cover should be prescribed. The patient may also have dry, inflamed eyes and the generous use of an ocular lubricant during anaesthesia is helpful.

Reference

1 Wills MH, Harris MM. *Anesthesiology*, 1987; **66:** 554–555.

Scleroderma

Systemic sclerosis, progressive systemic sclerosis,
CRST syndrome, CREST syndrome

Major problems
Airway and intubation difficulties
Impaired lung function
Difficulty with venous access
Prolonged sensory analgesia from local blocks

This disorder principally affects the skin, resulting in a widespread thickening and tightening. The appearance has been described as "waxy" and "leathery". The condition may range in severity from small localised areas of affected skin to generalised involvement of all organs in the body. Females are affected more than males and the peak incidence is in the fourth and fifth decades. The disease has a slowly progressive course and the patient may be on steroid therapy. The patient may in addition suffer from the CRST syndrome which consists of calcinosis, Raynaud's disease, scleroderma and telangiectasias.

Airway management may be a particular problem in these patients. The skin around the mouth tightens such that the mouth can hardly be opened. Intubation is therefore difficult and a fibreoptic technique may be needed. If telangiectasias are present in the mouth or nose as part of the CRST syndrome they may bleed profusely on minor trauma. Gastro-oesophageal sphincter incompetence together with abnormal oesophageal motility increases the risk of tracheal aspiration in these patients. Venous access is difficult and normal percutaneous techniques may be impossible. A cut down or central venous cannulation may be required. There is frequently impaired circulation to the limbs and the measurement of blood pressure may therefore be difficult. Doppler flow detectors are useful. Direct arterial cannulation should be avoided if possible because of the risk of further compromising circulation. The lungs are commonly involved in scleroderma. Interstitial fibrosis within the lungs together with reduced chest movement leads to a restrictive pattern of pulmonary impairment. Chest X-ray and lung function tests should be performed pre-operatively and the patient may need a period of postoperative controlled ventilation. Involvement of the heart may include pericarditis and conduction abnormalities and a pre-operative ECG is recommended. These patients may be relatively intravascularly hypovolaemic and so exaggerated falls in blood pressure can be produced by minimal vasodilatation. In long-standing cases pulmonary hypertension may develop and the use of a pulmonary flotation catheter may be appropriate [1]. The kidneys are often affected and it is wise to measure the urea and electrolytes pre-operatively. Gastrointestinal tract involvement impairs the absorption of certain substances, including vitamin K. A clotting screen should be performed. There are no particular general anaesthetic drugs or techniques which are contra-indicated. In view of the venous access problems it might seem convenient to use a gaseous induction technique. The other features of the condition, however, are such that intravenous access is desirable before the induction of anaesthesia. Co-existent Raynaud's disease is exacerbated by cold and local trauma and so a warm environment is recommended with warmed intravenous fluids. Irritant drugs, e.g. methohexitone, should not be injected into small peripheral veins [2]. Local and regional techniques have been used successfully in these patients. Difficulty may, however, be encountered with advancing the needle through the thickened tissues. Vasoconstrictors should be avoided. The duration of action of local anaesthetic agents is prolonged in scleroderma [3, 4]. The use of a Bier's block is not recommended [5].

References

1 Younker D, Harrison B. *Br. J. Anaesth.*, 1985; **57**: 1136−1139
2 Davidson-Lamb RW, Finlayson MCK. *Anaesthesia*, 1977; **32**: 893−895
3 Neill RS. *Br. J. Anaesth.*, 1980; **52**: 623−625.
4 Lewis GBH. *Can. Anaesth. Soc. J.*, 1974; **21**: 495−497.
5 Sweeney B. *Anaesthesia*, 1984; **39**: 1145.

Further reading

Smith GB, Shribman AJ. *Anaesthesia*, 1984; **39**: 443−455.
Thompson J. Conklin KA. *Anesthesiology*, 1983; **59**: 69−71.

Sheehan's syndrome

Major problems
Sensitive to barbiturates and opiates
Require peri-operative hydrocortisone therapy

Although pituitary infarction in Sheehan's syndrome classically occurs in the postpartum period, it may occur earlier in pregnancy. The result is a loss or severe reduction of all pituitary hormones. The patient thus appears pale and lethargic with loss of pubic and axillary hair and loss of libido. They may be hypotensive and complain of feeling cold.

In view of the adrenocortical insufficiency plasma electrolytes should be measured pre-operatively. The patent will lack the usual resistance to any stress, including that of surgery and anaesthesia. Treatment with hydrocortisone should be begun prior to anaesthesia. There is an increased sensitivity to barbiturates and opiates, which should be given in reduced dosage. If the pituitary dysfunction is of long standing then the patient is likely to be receiving replacement therapy with a number of hormones. These should be continued throughout the peri-operative period.

Further reading

Murray-Wilson, A. *Br. J. Anaesth.*, 1968; **40:** 996–998.

Shy-Drager syndrome

Major problems
Hypotension, especially with IPPV
Exaggerated hypertensive response to many
    sympathomimetic agents
Common autonomic indicators of anaesthetic
    depth are invalid
Absent tachycardic response to atropine

The Shy-Drager syndrome is characterised by progressive autonomic failure resulting from widespread degeneration of the autonomic nervous system and subsequently the central nervous system. Classically, postural hypotension (worse in mornings), reduction in sweating and sexual impotence are the principal symptoms. Other common complaints are dizziness or fainting, urinary symptoms, gastro-intestinal symptoms and other neurological manifestations, including neuropathies and Parkinsonism. Males are affected more often than females and the peak incidence is in the fifth to seventh decades.

When assessing these patients for anaesthesia it is useful to include some test of autonomic function. The fall in blood pressure on standing (exaggerated in Shy-Drager syndrome), rise in blood pressure in response to stress (reduced or absent in the Shy-Drager syndrome) and the heart rate and blood pressure changes in response to a Valsalva manoeuvre (reduced or absent in Shy-Drager syndrome) are all appropriate tests.

Hypotension is a common problem during anaesthesia. Intermittent positive pressure ventilation will usually produce marked hypotension in these patients. Anaesthetic agents which have a tendency to produce hypotension should be used with care; cyclopropane and diethyl ether suppress baroreceptor reflexes and should be avoided [1]. In order to prevent undue hypotension it is recommended that the circulating volume be kept well maintained [2]. Directly acting sympathomimetics, e.g. noradrenaline, methoxamine, phenylephrine, produce an exaggerated action and so should be given in reduced dosage. Indirectly acting sympathomimetics, e.g. ephedrine, frequently have no effect. There may be no response to atropine. Elastic stockings, calf compressors, or even a G-suit may also be helpful. The abnormal sympathetic responses make normal clinical measurement of the depth of anaesthesia more difficult because sweating, tachycardia and blood pressure changes may be absent. The mainstay of treatment at present is 9 alpha fludrocortisone and this should be continued throughout the peri-operative period [3]. Epidural anaesthesia has been successfully used. There is negligible fall in blood pressure from sympathetic blockade because the patients already have a reduced sympathetic tone.

References

1 Cohen CA. *Anesthesiology*, 1971; **35:** 95−97.
2 Bevan DR. *Anaesthesia*, 1979; **34:** 866−873.
3 Hutchinson RC, Sugden JC. *Anaesthesia*, 1984; **39:** 1229−1231.

Sick sinus syndrome

Major problem
Sudden cardiac arrest

A range of cardiac dysrhythmias resulting from malfunction of the atrial pacemaker are included under the term "Sick sinus syndrome". These include sinus bradycardia, sinus arrest and the bradycardia-tachycardia syndrome. It is usually a condition affecting the older age groups. It has a slow, insidious onset but may affect patients of any age. Association with diabetes, thyroid disease, congenital heart disease and ischaemic heart disease have all been suggested.

Pre-operative recognition of the syndrome is a problem. The case report referenced [1] described a patient who had a sudden cardiac arrest after 30 minutes of uneventful general anaesthesia. It was only by close questioning afterwards that a history of occasional dizzy spells was elicited. A history of dizziness or syncopal attacks should therefore arouse suspicion, but such events may be dismissed by the patient and not reported. The best treatment for the sick sinus syndrome is the insertion of a pacing wire. This may have to be later converted to a permanent implanted pacemaker. Atropine or isoprenaline may be used but their action is only temporary and the abnormal cardiac conduction system may be refractory to pharmacological treatment.

Reference

1 Burt DER. *Anaesthesia*, 1982; **37**: 1108−1111.

Sickle cell disease

Major problems
Avoid hypoxia, hypotension, hypovolaemia,
hypothermia, acidosis and venous stasis

This hereditary haemolytic anaemia mainly affects people whose background originated from Central and West Africa, West Indies and certain Mediterranean regions around Turkey, Greece and Italy. It is inherited in an autosomal recessive fashion, there being two subtypes, sickle cell disease (homozygous form—HbA almost entirely replaced by HbS) and sickle cell trait (heterozygous form—about 30–40% HbS, remainder HbA). In the homozygous form the abnormal haemoglobin molecule crystallises under the influence of moderate hypoxia resulting in distortion of the red blood cells (sickling) and haemolysis. These patients are also prone to develop capillary and venous thrombosis and are often anaemic. Sickling may occur in patients with sickle trait but not until the Po_2 has fallen to very low levels.

It is important that all patients whose racial background may include sickle cell disease are screened for this condition. The test is simple and straightforward. If for any reason the test cannot be performed, it is wise to treat all patients who could be at risk as having sickle cell disease until proved otherwise. The haemoglobin should also be measured. A moderate degree of anaemia is normal in these patients and should be accepted, replacing intra-operative losses as they occur. If the haemoglobin is very low (less than about 5 g dl^{-1}) [1, 2] then pre-operative transfusion should be undertaken. The principal factors to avoid are hypoxia, hypothermia, hypovolaemia, hypotension, circulatory stasis and acidosis. Appropriate management should therefore include preoxygenation and oxygen therapy for at least 24 hours postoperatively. Meticulous care is essential to avoid even transient hypoxia in these patients. The patient's temperature should be monitored and the use of a warm water circulating mattress on the operating table is helpful, with covers on all parts of the patient which do not need to be exposed. Careful attention should be paid to peri-operative fluid balance. The use of tourniquets for surgery and also Bier's block are contraindicated. The use of a constant infusion of bicarbonate or pre-operative administration of bicarbonate has been suggested but controversy surrounds its use and it is not generally employed. With the above exceptions, there are no contra-indications to any particular anaesthetic agent or technique, general or regional.

References

1 Howells TH, Huntsman RG, Boys JE, Mahmood A. *Br. J. Anaesth.*, 1972; **44**: 975−987.
2 Searle JF. *Anaesthesia*, 1973; **28**: 48−58.

Further reading

Browne RA. *Br. J. Anaesth.*, 1965; **37**: 181−188.
Gilbertson AA. *Br. J. Anaesth.*, 1965; **37**: 614−622.
Reithmuller R, Grundy EM, Radley-Smith R. *Anaesthesia*, 1982; **37**: 324−327.

Sjogren's syndrome

Keratoconjunctivitis sicca

Major problem
Possible airway difficulties

Sjogren's syndrome is characterised by pathological dryness of the mouth and eyes associated with inflammatory arthritis. The condition is probably auto-immune in origin, often being associated with other conditions of an auto-immune aetiology. Approximately 50% of patients with Sjogren's syndrome have rheumatoid arthritis. The reduction in secretions may affect other sites including the gastrointestinal tract, tracheobronchial tree and vaginal mucosa.

The fibrosis and inflammation of the lacrimal and salivary glands may result in considerable swelling. The enlargement of the parotid and submandibular glands may make it difficult to find a suitable facemask to fit the patient. Airway or intubation problems may also be encountered. Involvement of the tracheobronchial tree results in scanty viscid mucus with peripheral mucus plugging and an increased incidence of chest infections. Atropine, hyoscine and other drying agents should be avoided. It may be helpful to humidify the patient's inspired gases. A suitable ocular lubricant should be instilled into the eyes to prevent any further drying out.

Further reading

Isenberg D, Crisp A. *Hospital Update*, 1985; **11**: 273–283.

Sleep paralysis

Major problem
Postoperative stupor

Sleep paralysis is a state in which there is thought to be a dissociation between sensory and motor function — perhaps a dysfunction of the reticular activating system. The patient may be fully awake but totally unable to move. This state occurs most commonly on going to sleep or on waking. It is thought to have been experienced by about 5% of the population but is only clinically evident in a minority of sufferers.

The main problem is of the differential diagnosis in the post-operative period. Treatment with physostigmine (2 mg IV) will terminate the apparent stupor.

Further reading

Spector M, Bourke DL. *Anesthesiology*, 1977; **46**: 296−297

Spinal muscular atrophy
Infantile spinal muscular atrophy,
Werdnig-Hoffmann disease

Major problems
Increased sensitivity to anaesthetic agents,
respiratory depressants and muscle relaxants
Impaired airway protective reflexes

These are a group of hereditary spinal muscular atrophies, the common feature of all of them being selective degeneration of the anterior horn cells in the spinal cord and of the lower cranial nerve motor nuclei. Generalised muscle weakness and hypotonia result. Sensation is unaffected. If the bulbar muscles are affected then the airway protective reflexes will be compromised with subsequent episodes of tracheal aspiration. The muscular weakness also reduces respiratory reserve and there is frequently a co-existing kyphoscoliosis. The infantile form (Werdnig-Hoffmann disease) is more severe and sufferers do not usually survive beyond childhood.

Pre-operative preparation of these patients should include assessment of respiratory reserve. Premedication with morphine and hyoscine has been used [1]. The patients are sensitive to anaesthetic agents and so a reduced dosage of thiopentone or other induction agent will be required. Volatile anaesthetic agents are tolerated. Advice regarding the use of muscle relaxants is less clear. Suxamethonium theoretically is inadvisable due to the possibility of an exaggerated rise in plasma potassium (denervated muscle is present). It has, however, been used without problems [2]. There is likely to be an increased sensitivity to the non-depolarising relaxants and these should be given in a reduced dosage. Postoperatively the patients may be slower than expected in awakening. Ventilatory support may be needed. The tracheal tube should not be removed until the patient is fully awake and all airway protective reflexes have returned. The patients have an increased sensitivity to all respiratory depressant drugs.

References

1 Wislicki L. *Anaesthesia*, 1962; **17:** 482−487.
2 Seddon SJ. *Anaesthesia*,1985; **40:** 820−821.

Further reading

Ellis FR. *Br. J. Anaesth.*, 1974; **46:** 603−612.

Spondylometepiphyseal dysplasia

Major problems
Atlanto-axial instability
Intubating difficulties
Reduced respiratory reserve

This rare form of dwarfism is characterised by short limbs, kyphoscoliosis with compression of the spinal cord, odontoid hypoplasia, a contracted pelvis and hip deformities. There may be other associated congenital abnormalities, including cleft palate, heart lesions and kidney lesions. Spondylometepiphyseal dysplasia is not the same as spondyloepiphyseal dysplasia.

Airway management may be difficult in these patients and care must be taken with movements of the head on the neck due to the atlanto-axial instability. It may be wise to fit the patient with a comfortable rigid cervical collar pre-operatively to limit neck movement and to keep this *in situ* throughout. The kyphoscoliosis introduces potential for respiratory embarrassment. The functional residual capacity is reduced in dwarf patients and even more so in pregnant dwarf patients at term [1]. Hypoxaemia is therefore very likely to occur despite apparently adequate pre-oxygenation. Ketamine and suxamethonium were used satisfactorily in one patient [1]. There is no contra-indication to regional techniques although difficulty may be experienced because of the spinal deformity.

Reference

1 Benson KT, Dozier NJ, Goto H, Arakawa K. *Anesthesiology*, 1985; **63:** 548–550.

Sprengel's deformity

Major problems
Airway and intubation difficulties

In Sprengel's deformity hypoplastic scapulae are present which lie in a more superior position than normal, encroaching on the base of the neck. In addition, abnormalities of the cervical vertebrae may be present, including cervical ribs, fused vertebrae and other rib abnormalities. The end result is gross limitation of movement of one or both shoulders and grossly reduced or even absent ability to flex or extend the neck.

In the case referenced [1] the deformity was such that mouth opening was greatly limited, the neck was rigid and the trachea was impalpable. Furthermore, the trachea was seen on X-ray to be somewhat deviated from the normal position and thus intubation by any means other than a fibreoptic technique was considered impossible. Tracheostomy would also have been impossible. General anaesthesia was achieved using ketamine and maintained by repeated doses of ketamine. No problems were encountered.

Reference

1 Ruhomally H. *Br. J. Anaesth.*, 1976; **48**: 393.

Stiff baby syndrome

Hyperekplexia, startle disease

Major problem
Resistance to suxamethonium

This rare genetic abnormality is inherited in an autosomal dominant fashion. It is characterised by the appearance of increased muscle tone to the point where the patient is quite rigid. It begins immediately after birth and slowly disappears over the first few years of life. Patients are intellectually normal with a full life span. In addition, they respond to minor stimuli with an exaggerated startled response.

There is only one reported case of anaesthesia in a five-month-old baby with this disorder [1]. The patient was resistant to suxamethonium (2 mg kg^{-1} produced 74% neuromuscular blockade) although its duration of action was within normal limits. There was an overall additional increase in muscle tone following the suxamethonium and a negligible change in plasma potassium. The response to pancuronium and neostigmine was normal. The response to other drugs is not known although it has been postulated that opiates or nitrous oxide might make the rigidity worse and that benzodiazepines, barbiturates, ketanserin and volatile anaesthetic agents might attenuate the rigidity [2].

References

1 Cook WP, Kaplan RF. *Anesthesiology*, 1986; **65:**525−528.
2 Weinger MB. *Anesthesiology*, 1987; **66:** 580−581.

Sturge-Weber syndrome

Major problems
Airway and intubation difficulties

A unilateral angioma of the face is present (port wine stain), commonly with intracranial involvement. Epilepsy, mental retardation and glaucoma are also common findings and there may be a progressive neurological deficit together with hemiparesis.

Problems with anaesthesia are principally due to the physical presence of the facial angioma. Its size and site may produce airway and intubation difficulties. The vascular, hypertrophied tissues are bulky and may also bleed if traumatised. It is possible for the larynx and trachea to be involved in the angioma and so thereby make intubation hazardous.

Further reading

Aldridge LM. *Anaesthesia*, 1987; **42:** 1239–1240.

Subclavian steal syndrome

Major problem
Avoid hypocapnia

This syndrome results from blockage of the subclavian artery between its origin from the aorta and its bifurcation to form the vertebral artery. Blood flow to the arm is provided partly by collaterals and partly by retrograde flow back down the vertebral artery from the circle of Willis. Exercising that arm then increases flow down the vertebral artery stealing blood away from the base of the brain. The result is dizziness or fainting attacks when the affected arm is exercised.

In the case described [1] general anaesthesia was provided by conventional means without problems. It was noted that hypocapnia consequent upon hyperventilation resulted in an increase in flow to the affected arm. It is likely that this increased flow was at the expense of a reduced flow to the brain, a situation which may have serious consequences. It is therefore recommended that hypocapnia is avoided in these patients.

Reference

1 Thompson RJ. *Anaesthesia*, 1986; **41**: 1026–1028.

Systemic lupus erythematosis

Major problems
Arthritis in many joints
Steroid therapy

This autoimmune disorder affects women predominantly, with a peak incidence in the third decade. It is a multisystem disorder, although the most common clinical features are arthritis, myalgia, skin eruption, pyrexia, neurological and psychiatric disturbances. Other features include nephritis, pericarditis, myocarditis, anaemia, pleurisy, pleural effusions and gastro-intestinal upsets. The patient may be receiving steroid or immunosuppresant therapy.

Pre-operative assessment of these patients should include lung fuction tests, full blood count, urea and electrolytes. Increased peri-operative steroid cover may be required. There are no specific anaesthetic drugs or techniques which are contra-indicated. Intubation may be difficult if the arthritis affects the temporomandibular or crico-arytenoid joints. Arthritis in other joints may make positioning the patient a problem for certain procedures. If the patient is receiving immunosuppressant therapy then full sterile precautions must be taken with all instrumentation.

Further reading

Alfery DD, Benumof JL. In: *Anaesthesia and Uncommon Diseases: pathophysiologic and clinical correlations*, 2nd edn, 1981. Ed. Katz J, Benumof J, Kadis LB. WB Saunders, Philadelphia, pp. 240–244.

Takayasu's arteritis
Pulseless disease

Major problems
Absent pulses
Blood pressure measurement difficulty
Impaired blood flow to brain and other major
    organs

This chronic occlusive panarteritis affects young females mostly. It is a progressive disease beginning in the aorta and extending outwards to affect its branches. It principally involves vessels in the upper half of the body although any artery may be affected including the pulmonary arteries. Thickening of the arterial walls reduces arterial compliance and blood flow. The patients are often hypertensive and suffer thrombotic episodes in the affected arteries. They are often taking anticoagulants, antihypertensives and steroids.

Adequate cardiovascular monitoring is important in these patients but is a problem. Pulses are usually impalpable in the arms and possibly also in the legs. They should be detectable using Doppler flow probes and a combination of these with sphygmomanometer cuffs on arms and legs may be used for blood pressure monitoring. If arterial cannulation is desired then this will need to be performed by direct cutdown and not by a percutaneous technique. Two of the reported cases [1, 2] advocate the placement of a pulmonary flotation catheter before anaesthesia in view of the difficulties with other monitoring. No individual drugs or techniques have been reported to be contra-indicated. A thoracic epidural was used to good effect for post-operative analgesia in one case [1]. It is important that pre-operative cardiovascular medications be continued throughout. Steroid cover may be required. When performing tracheal intubation the head should not be extended too far because hyper-extension may stretch the carotid arteries and further compromise an already barely adequate flow. The renal vessels may be involved and so it is wise to assess renal function in the pre-operative period.

References

1 Thorburn JR, James MFM. *Anaesthesia*, 1986; **41:** 734–738.
2 Warner MA, Hughes DR, Messick JM. *Anesth. Analg.*, 1983; **62:** 532–535.

Further reading

Ramanathan S, Gupta U, Chalon J, Turndorf H. *Anesth. Analg.*, 1979; **58:** 247–249.

Testicular feminisation syndrome

Major problem
Small larynx

These patients are genotypically male (46 XY) but have an external appearance as of a normal female. There are no internal female genitalia but testes are usually present inside the abdomen.

The only reported anaesthesia for patients with the testicular feminisation syndrome notes the necessity for a smaller than expected tracheal tube. The larynx presumably retained its pre-pubertal size and 6.5 mm tubes were required for each of two patients, who were 18 and 21 years of age. General anaesthesia was otherwise uneventful. The patient may be unaware of his/her real genotype. It is therefore important not to enter into any conversation with the patient or relatives where this matter could be discussed.

Further reading

Sellers WFS, Yogendran S. *Anaesthesia*, 1987; **42:** 1243.

Thallassaemia

Cooley's anaemia

Major problems
Avoid hypoxia
Possible intubation difficulties

This abnormality of haemoglobin synthesis is inherited as an autosomal recessive condition with variable penetrance. It is most common around the Mediterranean coast, in Central Africa and Asia. There are a number of subtypes in existence but the two main subdivisions are thallassaemia major (homozygous form) and thallassaemia minor (heterozygous form). It is the major form which is the more serious and these patients may have moderate to severe anaemia with a shortened red cell life span.

Patients with thallassaemia minor should present no problems for anaesthesia. The following refers to thallassaemia major. It is wise to perform haemoglobin electrophoresis in these patients to check for other haemoglobin abnormalities, e.g. HBS thallassaemia. The haemoglobin level should be measured and, if low, pre-operative transfusion may be needed. It is essential to avoid even a transient period of hypoxaemia in these patients. They should receive pre-oxygenation at induction of anaesthesia and increased inspired oxygen in the postoperative period. A problem with intubation has been described secondary to hypertrophy of bones [1]. Hypertrophy of the maxilla made intubation difficult. There are no particular drugs or techniques which are contra-indicated in these patients.

Reference

1 Orr D. *Br. J. Anaesth.*, 1967; **39**: 585–586.

Thrombocytopaenic purpuras

Idiopathic thrombocytopaenic purpura,
autoimmune thrombocytopaenia,
thrombotic thrombocytopaenic purpura,
Moschkowitz disease, Felty's syndrome

Major problem
Increased bleeding tendency

A decrease in the number of platelets leads to spontaneous bleeding. This may present as bruising after minor trauma, gastro-intestinal haemorrhage, epistaxis or menorrhagia. Idiopathic thrombocytopaenic purpura is probably hereditary. Platelet anti-bodies are present and an acute exacerbation may be triggered by an acute viral infection. Secondary thrombocytopaenic pur-pura results form bone marrow dysfunction (see page 34); thrombotic thrombocytopaenic purpura mainly affects young women and is associated with neurological signs and renal damage.

Clotting screen, haemoglobin estimation and platelet count should be performed pre-operatively. Blood and platelet trans-fusions may both be required and it is wise to consult a haema-tologist for advice at this stage. If renal damage may be present renal function should be assessed pre-operatively and drugs which rely on the kidneys for excretion avoided. There are no contra-indications to general anaesthesia except that care must be taken with positioning and instrumentation because of the bleeding tendency. Local and regional blocks may be best avoided in view of the risk of haematoma formation. Hypertensive epi-sodes may put the patient at risk form subarachnoid haemor-rhage. In the case referenced [1] a caesarean section was performed instead of allowing normal labour. The patient may be receiving long term steroid therapy and, if so, increased peri-operative steroid cover should be considered.

Reference

1 Angiulo JP, Temple JT, Corrigan JJ, Galindo JH. *Anesthesiology*, 1977; **46**: 145–147.

Torsion dystonia

Dystonia musculorum deformans, Hallervorden-Spatz disease

Major problems
Possible airway/intubation problems
Contractures and abnormal postures make
  positioning difficult

Torsion dystonia is a progressive neurological disorder with a wide spectrum of appearances. There are two types, one inherited in an autosomal dominant fashion and the other autosomal recessive. Hallervorden-Spatz disease is an autosomally recessive inherited disorder of the basal ganglia which is very similar in appearance to torsion dystonia.

These conditions are characterised by abnormal sustained posturings of almost any part of the body which are exacerbated by stress and are reduced or disappear during sleep. The sustained nature of the posturings results in eventual muscle fibrosis and shortening and the deformities become fixed. The progressive nature of the disorder eventually results in severe disability for the patient.

In preparation of these patients for anaesthesia a thorough pre-operative evaluation of the patient with respect to posture is necessary. Relaxation of muscle spasm follows the induction of general anaesthesia but permanent contractures may be present. If these affect the jaw muscles or cervical spine airway management may be made difficult. Awake intubation has been advocated but in some patients noxious stimulation exacerbates the spasms. General anaesthesia with diazepam premedication, thiopentone and volatile agents has been safely used. The non-depolarising muscle relaxants may also be safely used. Denervated muscle may be present and so suxamethonium is theoretically inadvisable because of the risk of a hyperkalaemic response. It has, however, been used without problem. In the postoperative period the tracheal tube should be left *in situ* until the patient is fully awake. Any long-term treatment or medication should be continued throughout the peri-operative period.

Further reading

Davis NL, Davis R. *Anesthesiology*, 1975; **42**: 630−631.
Roy RC, McLain S, Wise A, Shaffner LdeS. *Anesthesiology*, 1983; **58**: 382−384.
Walajahi FH, Karasic LH. *Anesth. Analg.*, 1984; **63**: 616−618.

Tourette syndrome

Gilles de la Tourette syndrome

Major problem
Behavioural difficulties

Manifestations of this complex neuropsychiatric disturbance of childhood are principally behavioural. The patients show features of echolalia, coprolalia, tics, jerking movements and compulsive activity. Exacerbations may be precipitated by stress. They may be on a number of medications, in particular butyrophenones.

The most important consideration in these patients is the pre-operative visit. It is important to spend time talking to the patient to gain his or her confidence in addition to discussing the problems with the parents. A suitable sedative premedicant may be prescribed and the patient's normal pre-operative drug therapy must be continued throughout the peri-operative period. Care must be taken not to confuse the tics and movements with fits postoperatively. One case is reported [1] of a patient whose exacerbations were triggered by exposure to perfume and other aromatic substances. An uneventful anaesthetic was performed in this patient using halothane.

Reference

1 Morrison JF, Lockhart CH. *Anesth. Analg.*, 1986; **65:** 200–202.

Tracheal reconstruction

Tracheal cylindroma

Major problems
Complex airway management and intubation
difficulties

Reasons for tracheal reconstructive surgery include trauma, intratracheal tumours and congenital disorders of the trachea. Tracheal
tumours often present with stridor and dyspnoea. Severe congenital disorders are incompatible with life; less severe ones
require surgery in the neonatal period.

It is most important to carefully assess the patient pre-operatively with respect to the precise location of the lesion in the
trachea. If dyspnoea is a problem due to turbulent air flow
around an intratracheal lesion then breathing 80% helium, 20%
oxygen mixture may be helpful. Great care must be taken when
considering sedation, lest complete airway obstruction results.
The most important factor in these patients is airway management. Laryngoscopy and insertion of the tracheal tube through
the cords should not present a problem. The temptation to simply
go ahead with this technique must be resisted, however, because
it may be found to be impossible to advance the tube down the
trachea. If the lesion is low in the trachea, then it may be
possible to position a tube above the lesion. If it is high, then
either a small diameter armoured tube may be advanced past the
lesion (preferably under bronchoscopic control) or a low tracheostomy may be possible under local anaesthesia. The blind,
forceful insertion of a tube past the tumour is inadvisable as
trauma and bleeding may result. In one case [1], a rigid bronchoscope was inserted past the tumour and then left *in situ* for
ventilation during the first part of the surgery. In another, a
modified Foley catheter was used [2]. Whichever technique is
chosen, it should be either performed under local anaesthesia or
the patient anaesthetised spontaneously breathing a volatile
agent until the airway is secure.

During resection of the trachea the easiest method is for the surgeon to insert a cuffed tube into one main bronchus and then to connect this to the anaesthetic ventilator by means of a sterile anaesthetic circuit passing over the surgical field. In the latter stages of the reconstruction the surgeon's temporary bronchial tube has to be removed and a new tube advanced down the trachea to beyond the site of the anastomosis. Postoperatively patients should be extubated or the cuff of the tube deflated to minimise trauma on the suture line. If the trachea has been shortened it may be necessary to maintain the neck in acute flexion for some time by suturing the chin to the chest. This makes nursing and secretion control difficult. Additional methods of managing these cases are jet ventilation and extra-corporeal membrane oxygenation, both of which require specialised equipment and may also introduce additional problems.

References

1 Pollard BJ, Harrison MJ. *Eur. J. Anaesth.*, 1985; **2:** 387−394.
2 Abou-Madi MN, Cuadrado L, Domb B, Barnes J, Trop D. *Can. Anaes. Soc. J.*, 1979; **26:** 26−28.

Further reading

Ellis RH, Hinds CJ, Gadd LT. *Anaesthesia*, 1976; **31:** 1076−1080.
Heifitz M. *Anaesthesia*, 1974; **29:** 760−761.
Kamvyssi-Dea S, Kritikou P, Exarhos N, Skalkeas G. *Br. J. Anaesth.*, 1975; **47:** 82−84.
Lippmann M, Mok MS. *Br. J. Anaesth.*, 1977; **49:** 383−386.
Machell ES. *Br. J. Anaesth.*, 1977; **49:** 951.
Macnaughton FI. *Br. J. Anaesth.*, 1975; **47:** 1225−1227.
James OF, Moor PG. *Anaesth. Intensive Care*, 1983; **11:** 59−61.

Tracheobronchopathica osteochondroplastica

Major problem
Usually none

This rare condition is characterised by the appearance of submucosal protuberances within the lumen of the trachea or main bronchi. The outgrowths consist of bone or cartilage and are very slow growing. Diagnosis is usually made as an incidental finding at autopsy. The condition is usually asymptomatic but may give rise to voice changes, dyspnoea, dry cough, haemoptysis and recurrent pulmonary infections.

The only reported anaesthetic problem [1] is that of difficulty in advancing an endotracheal tube down the trachea.

Reference

1 Wagner RB, Barson PK. *Anesthesiology*, 1979; **51**: 269–270.

Tracheomegaly

Tracheobronchiomegaly, tracheobronchial malacia

Major problems
Walls of major airways prone to collapse
Increased risk of tracheal aspiration

Defects in the cartilagenous supports or the elastic and muscle fibres in the walls of the trachea and bronchi result in weakness of these structures. They are prone to collapse under the influence of increased intrathoracic pressure. In addition the soft tracheal walls are easily deformed and often dilate. The patients also have an increased tendency for tracheal aspiration. Tracheomalacia may be associated with an increased incidence of oesophageal atresia and tracheo-oesophageal fistula.

It may be difficult to obtain a good airtight seal using a conventional cuffed tracheal tube and this may further damage the softened trachea. The use of a pharyngeal pack may be necessary to ensure an airtight seal. A technique using high frequency ventilation has been suggested [1]. Care should be taken with the use of bronchial suction catheters lest the thinned walls are traumatised. The advantage of continuous positive airways pressure has been pointed out in these patients in an effort to splint the airways open [2] although a mechanical splint (tracheal stent) may on occasion be needed [3]. These patients have a weak cough reflex and so should be extubated in the lateral position with full precautions to prevent tracheal aspiration.

References

1 Smith GA, Castresana MR, Mandel SD. *Anesth. Analg.*, 1983; **62:** 538–539.
2 Kanter RK, Pollack MM, Wright WW, Grundfast KM. *Anesthesiology*, 1982; **57:** 54–56.
3 Page BA, Klein EF. *Anesthesiology*, 1977; **47:** 300–301.

Further reading

Parris WCV, Johnson AC. *Anesthesiology*, 1982; **56:** 141–143.

Transplanted heart

Major problems
Strict asepsis essential
Avoid hypotension
Increased likelihood of arrhythmias

Transplanted hearts do not behave exactly like normal hearts with respect to physiological and pharmacological responses. The transplanted hearts do not become re-innervated with an autonomic supply. They are therefore effectively denervated. The response to changes in preload (Starling's law) should be normal. Changes in cardiac output, e.g. following stress, take place principally by changes in stroke volume in response to circulating humoral mediators. This contrasts with a normal heart where rapid changes in rate are seen which are under the direct control of the autonomic nervous system. The response to exogenous catecholamines is normal. Atropine, digoxin, neostigmine and pancuronium, however, have no direct effect on the heart rate. The patient may have an implanted pacemaker.

These patients may be on treatment with a number of long-term medications. These usually include steroids, immunosuppressants, diuretics, anticoagulants and antiplatelet agents. With the possible exception of the anticoagulant and antiplatelet agents these should all be continued throughout the peri-operative period. The immunosuppressant therapy makes the patients exceedingly prone to all sorts of infection. Full asepsis is therefore essential for every procedure, including intubation, and it is wise to keep these to a minimum. Continuous ECG monitoring is essential because there is an increased likelihood of cardiac arrhythmias. The altered physiological situation makes the transplanted heart particularly sensitive to changes in intravascular volume. This must be well maintained and any falls in blood pressure treated immediately. Monitoring of the central venous pressure is valuable if more than a minimum blood loss is expected.

Further reading

Bricker SRW, Sugden JC. *Br. J. Anaesth.*, 1985; **57:** 634−637.
Samuels SI, Kanter SF. *Br. J. Anaesth.*, 1977; **49:** 265−268.

Trisomy 21

Down's syndrome, mongolism

Major problems

Associated congenital heart disease

Atlanto-axial instability

Possible intubation problems

The presence of an additional chromosome 21 leads to multiple malformations, mental and growth retardation. Clinical features include oblique palpebral fissures with epicanthic folds, small maxilla and mandible with large tongue, high arched palate and underdeveloped larynx. Congenital cardiac lesions are present in 40% of these patients and atlanto-axial instability in 20%. Although mentally retarded they usually have a docile friendly nature.

In the pre-operative assessment of these patients a high index of suspicion must be maintained for the presence of congenital heart lesions. Antibiotic prophylaxis against bacterial endocarditis may be required. Unless the patient has a proven stable atlanto-axial joint it is wise to treat all these patients as though they have such instability and take great care when moving and positioning the head and neck. Although they have a small mouth and large tongue intubation is not usually a great problem. The small larynx may need a tube of a smaller diameter than otherwise expected. There are no specific anaesthetic drugs or techniques which are contra-indicated. Reports have suggested that they are sensitive to the chronotropic effect of atropine but this is disputed. Difficulties may be encountered with excess salivation and larger than normal doses of hyoscine may be required to depress salivation.

Further reading

Moore RA, McNicholas KW, Warran SP. *Anesth. Analg.*, 1987; **66**: 89–90.

Morray JP, MacGillivray R, Duker G. *Anesthesiology*, 1986; **65**: 221–224.

Wark HJ, Overton JH, Marian P. *Anaesthesia*, 1983; **38**: 871–874.

Williams JP, Somerville GM, Miner ME, Reilly D. *Anesthesiology*, 1987; **67**: 253–254.

Turner's syndrome

Major problems
Difficult intubation
Congenital heart lesions
Impaired renal function

These patients are phenotypically female but genotypically XO. The resulting appearance is of short stature with a short webbed neck. Secondary sexual characteristics are either absent or under-developed. There is an association with other congenital abnormalities, especially coarctation of the aorta, cardiac valvular lesions and renal anomalies.

The short webbed neck may make intubation difficult in these patients. Full precautions in anticipation of a difficult intubation are therefore important. In addition, once intubation is accomplished, care must be taken not to advance the tracheal tube into one main bronchus because of the very short trachea. The possibility of co-existent congenital heart disease must be borne in mind during the pre-operative assessment of these patients and patient management appropriate to the disorder instituted. Antibiotic prophylaxis against bacterial endocarditis should be considered. In view of the high incidence of co-existing renal disorders and the likelihood of impaired renal function the action of renally excreted drugs will probably be prolonged. These drugs should be avoided or given with care in reduced dosage.

Further reading

Divekar VM, Kothari MD, Kamder BM. *Can. Anaesth. Soc. J.*, 1983; **30**: 417–418.

Von Hippel-Lindau disease

Cerebelloretinal haemangioblastosis

Major problem
Avoid hypotensive episodes

This disorder is inherited in an autosomal dominant fashion. It is characterised by the presence of angiomas in the retina, central nervous system and occasionally viscera. It has also been linked with phaeochromocytoma and kidney and liver disorders, but the associations are uncommon.

Anaesthetic considerations relate principally to any other underlying pathology present. Intracerebral angiomas may bleed and so hypertensive episodes should be avoided if possible. In the reference cited [1], it was felt inadvisable to allow a pregnant woman with Von Hippel-Lindau disease to proceed with a normal labour. Elective caesarean section was performed under epidural anaesthesia without problems. Syntocinon was used instead of ergometrine.

Reference

1 Matthews AJ, Halshaw J. *Anaesthesia*, 1986; **41:** 853−855.

Von Willebrand's disease

Pseudohaemophilia

Major problem
Increased bleeding

This disorder of Factor VIII synthesis shows a bleeding pattern more characteristic of a platelet defect than does haemophilia (see page 100). It is inherited in an autosomal dominant manner with a variable expressivity. In addition to the Factor VIII deficiency there is an associated decreased platelet function and possibly a capillary abnormality. The result is a prolonged bleeding time.

Any surgery may be a problem and it is wise to seek the advice of a haematologist regarding peri-operative management of the bleeding disorder. Administration of Factor VIII concentrate is usually needed. Treatment with tranexamic acid and desmopressin may reduce the requirement for clotting factor replacement. There are no specific anaesthetic agents or techniques which are contra-indicated in these patients. They do bleed markedly following minor episodes of trauma and so intubation, pharyngeal suction, venepuncture and positioning of the patient must all be done with great care. Regional nerve blocks should be avoided as should intramuscular injections.

Further reading

Bowes JB. *Br. J. Anaesth.*, 1969; **41**: 894–897.

Weaver's syndrome

Major problem
Difficult intubation

This rare developmental condition is characterised by accelerated growth beginning in the prenatal period. There is advanced growth and osseous maturation leading to an adult sized head with a small jaw, large tongue and receding chin. The patients have an unusual craniofacial appearance.

The principal problem is one of intubation difficulty. In the case referenced [1] there was no difficulty with maintaining the airway with a facemask. The larynx could not be seen, however, on direct laryngoscopy and as intubation was not needed it was not attempted. When preparing for anaesthesia in these patients all possible precautions for the difficult intubation must be taken. It may be necessary to use a fibreoptic instrument. It is not known how the larynx is affected by the growth abnormalities and so a range of sizes of tubes should be prepared.

Reference

1 Turner DR, Downing JW. *Br. J. Anaesth.*, 1985; **57**: 1260–1263.

Wiskott-Aldrich syndrome

Major problems
Strict asepsis necessary for all procedures
Bleeding tendency

The combination of thrombocytopaenia with eczema and with recurrent infections makes the Wiskott-Aldrich syndrome. It is inherited in an X-linked recessive manner and therefore only affects males. Anaemia, epistaxis, splenomegaly and episodes of bloody diarrhoea are common findings. The patients are very susceptible to all forms of infection, in particular herpes simplex, and usually die from overwhelming infection in early adulthood.

The most important anaesthetic consideration in these patients is the prevention of infection. Strict asepsis is necessary for all procedures, including intubation and venepuncture. Any pre-existing infection must also be treated before surgery. Thrombocytopaenia and anaemia may require pre-operative transfusion of both platelets and red cells. The advice of the haematologist should be sought because irradiated blood may be necessary to prevent a graft versus host reaction. There are no specific contra-indications to general anaesthesia but regional blockade may be inadvisable in view of the low platelet count.

Further reading

Ravin MB. *Anesthesiology*, 1966; **27**: 199–201.

Wolff-Parkinson-White syndrome

Pre-excitation syndrome, Lown-Ganong-Levine syndrome

Major problem
Sudden tachyarrhythmias

There is an anomalous atrioventricular conduction pathway in the Wolff-Parkinson-White syndrome along which electrical impulses may travel allowing premature excitation of the ventricles. In addition, this pathway may conduct impulses in a retrograde manner allowing premature atrial contraction. If this electrical loop, or re-entry loop, begins to function repetitively a supraventricular tachycardia results. The characteristic ECG appearance is of a short PR interval with a widened QRS complex containing a delta wave in the upstroke of the R wave.

The Lown-Ganong-Levine syndrome also possesses an anomalous atrioventricular conduction pathway but here a more common arrhythmia is fast atrial flutter/fibrillation. The PR interval is shortened but the QRS complex appears normal.

During the tachycardic episodes the patient may faint or may develop angina or cardiac failure. ST and T wave changes may also appear, which are very similar to those of acute myocardial ischaemia, making difficulties in interpretation and diagnosis.

The most important anaesthetic consideration in these patients is the prevention of tachyarrhythmias. These are favoured by sympathetic stimulation and anxiety. It is much easier to prevent the arrhythmias than to treat them once they are established. A good sedative premedicant is helpful. Any agent which has a tendency to produce a tachycardia, e.g. atropine or gallamine, should be avoided. Various anaesthetic regimes have been proposed for these patients, including strict neurolept anaesthesia and also the use of volatile agents, all without difficulty. It is likely therefore that no particular anaesthetic agent is contraindicated and that the important considerations are maintaining an adequate depth of anaesthesia and preventing hypotension, which itself may give rise to a compensatory tachycardia. If a tachyarrhythmia does arise then the following may be tried:

carotid sinus massage, procainamide, propranolol, quinidine, edrophonium, phenylephrine, amiodorone. The two agents verapamil and lignocaine have been reported both to terminate a tachyarrhythmia and also to induce a tachyarrhythmia and so are best avoided. Synchronised DC cardioversion may also be effective in terminating an arrhythmia in some instances.

Further reading

Campkin TV, Moore KP. *Br. J. Anaesth.*, 1969; **41:** 274–276.
Caramella JP, Malbezin S, Couderc E, Berger JL, Desmonts JM. *Can. Anaesth. Soc. J.*, 1983; **30:** 185–190.
Hannington-Kiff JG. *Br. J. Anaesth.*, 1968; **40:** 791–795.
Jacobson L, Turnquist K, Masley S. *Anaesthesia*, 1985; **40:** 657–660.
Sadowski AR, Moyers JR. *Anesthesiology*, 1979; **51:** 553–556.
Van der Starre PJA. *Anesthesiology*, 1978; **48:** 369–372.

Index

3rd and 4th arch syndrome *see* DiGeorge syndrome

5p deletion syndrome *see* Cri du chat syndrome

Abdominal muscular deficiency syndrome *see* Prune belly syndrome

Acanthosis nigricans 1

Achondroplasia 2–3

Acid maltase deficiency *see* Glycogen storage disease II

Acromegaly 4–5

Acute idiopathic polyneuritis 6–7

Acute infectious polyneuritis *see* Acute idiopathic polyneuritis

Adenomatosis, multiple endocrine *see* Apudomas

Albers-Schonberg disease *see* Osteopetrosis

Alpha glucosidase deficiency *see* Glycogen storage disease II

Alveolar proteinosis 8–9

Amaurosis congenita 10

Amelia 11

American trypanosomiasis 12

Amyloidosis 13

Amyotrophic lateral sclerosis 14–15

Anaemia *see* Bone marrow failure

Analgesia – congenital 16

Angina, Ludwig's *see* Ludwig's angina

Angina, Prinzmetal's *see* Prinzmetal's variant angina

Angioedema, hereditary *see* Hereditary angioedema

Ankylosing spondylitis 17

Anomalous lung 18

Aortic arch abnormalities 19

Apnoea – obstructive sleep 20–21

Apudomas 22–23

Arachnodactyly 24

Arthrogryposis multiplex congenita 25

Asymmetrical septal hypertrophy 26

Athlete's heart 27

Auto erythrocyte sensitisation syndrome 28

Autoimmune thrombocytopaenia *see* Thrombocytopaenic purpura

Autonomic dysfunction *see* Dysautonomia

Autonomic hyperreflexia 29

Bartter's syndrome 30

Behçet's syndrome 31

Bilirubin metabolism – abnormalities 32–33

Bone marrow failure 34–35

Branched chain ketonuria 36

Broad Thumb-Hallux syndrome *see* Rubenstein-Taybi syndrome

Buerger's disease 37

Bullous lung disease 38–39

Burkitt's lymphoma *see* Lymphoma

Camarati-Engelmann disease *see* Engelmann's disease

Carcinoid syndrome 40

Cardioauditory syndrome *see* Prolonged QT Syndrome

Carnitine myopathy *see* Myopathy – carnitine deficiency

Cat cry syndrome *see* Cri du chat

Central alveolar hypoventilation *see* Apnoea – obstructive sleep

Central core disease *see* Muscular dystrophy

Cerebelloretinal haemangioblastosis *see* Von Hippel-Lindau disease

Cerebrovascular Moya Moya disease *see* Moya Moya disease

Chagas' disease *see* American trypanosomiasis

Charcot-Marie-Tooth Disease *see* Peroneal muscular atrophy

Chemodectoma *see* Glomus jugulare

Cherubism 41

Cholinesterase deficiency 42

Chondrodystrophia calcificans congenita 43

Chondrodystrophia fetalis *see* Achondroplasia

Chondroectodermal dysplasia *see* Dwarfism
Chondro-osteodystrophy *see* Mucopolysaccharidosis IV
Christmas disease *see* Haemophilia
Chronic lymphoedema 44
Coarctation of aorta 45
Cockayne's syndrome 46
Congenital complete heart block 47
Congenital facial diplegia *see* Facial diplegia (congenital)
Congenital myasthenia gravis *see* Myasthenia gravis
Conjoined twins 48–49
Conn's syndrome *see* Hyperaldosteronism
Conradi's syndrome *see* Chondrodystrophia calcificans congenita
Cooley's anaemia *see* Thallassaemia
Corpus callosum (agenesis) 50
Cranio-carpal-tarsal dysplasia *see* Freeman-Sheldon syndrome
Crest syndrome *see* Scleroderma
Cretinism *see* Hypothyroidism
Creutzfeldt-Jakob disease 51
Cri du chat syndrome 52
Crigler-Najjar syndrome *see* Bilirubin metabolism — abnormalities
CRST syndrome *see* Scleroderma
Cushing's syndrome 53–54
Cystic fibrosis 55–56
Cystic hygroma 57
Cystinosis *see* Fanconi syndrome

de Toni Fanconi syndrome *see* Fanconi syndrome
Deleted (5P) syndrome *see* Cri du chat syndrome
Demyelinating disorders *see* Multiple sclerosis
Denervation hypersensitivity 58
Dermatomyositis 59
Diabetic gastroparesis *see* Gastroparesis (diabetic)
DiGeorge syndrome 60
Disseminated sclerosis *see* Multiple sclerosis
Distal muscular dystrophy 61
Down's syndrome *see* Trisomy 21
Dubin Johnson syndrome *see* Bilirubin metabolism — abnormalities

Duchenne muscular dystrophy *see* Muscular dystrophy
Dutch-Kentucky syndrome 62
Dwarfism 63–64
Dysautonomia 65–66
Dysplasia epiphysalis punctata *see* Chondrodystrophia calcificans congenita
Dystonia musculorum deformans *see* Torsion dystonia
Dystrophia myotonica *see* Myotonica dystrophia

Eaton-Lambert syndrome *see* Myasthenic syndrome
Ebstein's anomaly 67–68
Ectromelia *see* Amelia
Ehlers-Danlos syndrome 69
Eisenmenger syndrome 70–71
Ellis-van Creveld disease *see* Chondroectodermal dysplasia
Endocrine adenomatosis (multiple) *see* Apudomas
Engelmann's disease 72
Eosinophilic myositis 73
Epidermolysis bullosa 74–76
Epidermolysis bullosa dystrophica *see* Epidermolysis bullosa
Epiphyseal dysplasia, multiple *see* Dwarfism
Erythema multiforme 77
Eulenberg's disease *see* Paramyotonia congenita
Exomphalos 78

Face — chronic lymphoedema *see* Chronic lymphoedema of face
Facial diplegia (congenital) 79
Fairbank's disease *see* Dwarfism
Familial dysautonomia *see* Dysautonomia
Familial hyperkalaemic periodic paralysis *see* Familial periodic paralysis
Familial hypokalaemic periodic paralysis *see* Familial periodic paralysis
Familial periodic paralysis 80
Fanconi syndrome 81
Favism *see* Glucose 6-phosphate dehydrogenase deficiency
Felty's syndrome *see* Thrombocytopaenia purpura
Fetal alcohol syndrome 82

Fragilitans ossium *see* Osteogenesis imperfecta
Freeman-Sheldon syndrome 83
Friedreich's ataxia 84
Fructose-1, 6-diphosphatase deficiency 85
Fused jaws 86

G-syndrome *see* Opitz Frias syndrome
Gardner's syndrome 87
Gastroparesis (diabetic) 88
Gilbert's syndrome *see* Bilirubin metabolism — abnormalities
Gilles de la Tourette syndrome *see* Tourette syndrome
Glomus jugulare 89–90
Glossopharyngeal neuralgia 91
Glucagonoma 92
Glucose 6-phosphatase deficiency *see* Glycogen storage disease I
Glucose 6-phosphate dehydrogenase deficiency 93
Glycogen storage disease I 94
Glycogen storage disease II 95–96
Glycogen storage disease V 97
Glycogen storage disease IX 98
Goldenhars syndrome *see* Oculo-auriculovertebral dysplasia
Groenblad-Strandberg syndrome *see* Pseudoxanthoma elasticum
Guillain-Barré syndrome *see* Acute idiopathic polyneuritis

Haemolytic uraemic syndrome 99
Haemophilia a and b 100
Hallerman-Streiff syndrome 101
Hallervorden-Spatz disease *see* Torsion dystonia
Heart — athlete's *see* Athlete's heart
Heart block 102
Heart block — congenital complete *see* Congenital complete heart block
Heart — denervated *see* Transplanted heart
Heart — transplanted *see* Transplanted heart
Heerfordts syndrome 103
Hepatic storage disease *see* Bilirubin metabolism — abnormalities
Hereditary angioedema 104
Heredopathia atactica polyneuritiformis 105

Hippopotamus face 106
Hodgkin's disease *see* Lymphoma
Hoffman's disease *see* Myotonica dystrophia
Homocystinuria 107
Hunters disease *see* Mucopolysaccharidosis II
Huntington's chorea 108
Hurler-Sheie's disease *see* Mucopolysaccharidosis I S
Hurler's syndrome *see* Mucopolysaccharidosis I H
Hutchinson-Gilford syndrome *see* Progeria
Hyperaldosteronism 109–110
Hypercalcaemia 111–112
Hypercholinesterasaemia 113
Hypereosinophilic syndrome 114
Hyperparathyroidism *see* Hypercalcaemia
Hyperreflexia — autonomic *see* Autonomic hyperreflexia
Hyperekplexia *see* Stiff baby syndrome
Hyperinsulinism 115
Hyperlipoproteinaemia 116
Hypermagnesaemia 117
Hyperreninism 118
Hyperthyroidism 119
Hypophosphataemia 120
Hypospadias-dysphagia syndrome *see* Opitz Frias syndrome
Hypothyroidism 121

Idiopathic hypertrophic subaortic stenosis *see* Asymmetrical septal hypertrophy
Idiopathic pulmonary haemosiderosis 122
Idiopathic thrombocytopenic purpura *see* Thrombocytopaenic purpura
Infantile lobar emphysema 123
Infantile spinal muscular atrophy *see* Spinal muscular atrophy
Infectious mononucleosis 124
Insulinoma *see* Apudomas

Jakob-Creutzfeldt disease *see* Creutzfeldt-Jakob disease
Jaw winking syndrome 125
Jaws — fibro-osseous dysplasia *see* Hippopotamus face
Jaws — hereditary fibrous dysplasia

see Cherubism
Jervell-Lange-Nielson syndrome *see*
Prolonged QT syndrome
Juvenile chronic polyarthritis   126

Kawasaki disease   127
Kearns Sayer syndrome *see*
Ophthalmoplegia plus
Keratoconjunctivitis sicca *see*
Sjogren's syndrome
Klippel-Feil syndrome   128

Lactic acidosis *see* Pyruvate
dehydrogenase deficiency
Larsen's syndrome   129
Laryngeal papillomatosis   130
Laryngocoele   131
Laryngotrache-oesophageal cleft
132–133
Leber's disease *see* Amaurosis
congenita
Leigh's syndrome   134
Lesch-Nyhan syndrome   135
Leucopaenia *see* Bone marrow
failure
Lignac-Fanconi syndrome *see*
Fanconi syndrome
Long QT syndrome *see* Prolonged QT
syndrome
Lown-Ganong-Levine syndrome *see*
Wolff-Parkinson-White syndrome
Ludwig's angina   136–137
Lung—anomalous *see* Anomalous
lung
Lymphoedema—chronic facial *see*
Chronic lymphoedema of face
Lymphoma   138–139
Lymphosarcoma cutis   140

Malignant hyperpyrexia   141–143
Mandibulofacial dysostosis   144–
145
Maple-syrup urine disease *see*
Branched chain ketonuria
Marble bone disease *see*
Osteopetrosis
Marcus Gunn syndrome *see* Jaw
winking syndrome
Marfan's syndrome *see*
Arachnodactyly
Marie Strumpell arthritis *see*
Ankylosing spondylitis
Maroteaux-Lamy syndrome *see*
Mucopolysaccharidosis VI

Mass reflex *see* Autonomic
hyperreflexia
Mastocytosis   146–147
McArdle's disease *see* Glycogen
storage disease V
Meig's syndrome   148
Metaphyseal dysostosis *see* Dwarfism
Metastatic calcific cardiomyopathy
see Metastatic myocardial
calcification
Metastatic myocardial calcification
149
Methaemoglobinaemia   150–151
Mitral valve prolapse   152–153
Mobius syndrome *see* Facial diplegia
(congenital)
Moebius syndrome *see* Facial diplegia
(congenital)
Mongolism *see* Trisomy   21
Morbid obesity *see* Obesity
Morquio's syndrome *see*
Mucopolysaccharidosis IV
Moschkowitz disease *see*
Thrombocytopaenic purpura
Motor neurone disease *see*
Amyotrophic lateral sclerosis
Moya Moya disease   154
Mucocutaneous lymph node
syndrome *see* Kawasaki disease
Mucopolysaccharidosis I H   155–
156
Mucopolysaccharidosis IHS *see*
Mucopolysaccharidosis I S
Mucopolysaccharidosis I S   157
Mucopolysaccharidosis II   158
Mucopolysaccharidosis III   159
Mucopolysaccharidosis IV   160–
161
Mucopolysaccharidosis V *see*
Mucopolysaccharidosis I S
Mucopolysaccharidosis VI   162
Multiple endocrine adenomatosis *see*
Apudomas
Multiple sclerosis   163–164
Muscle glycogen phosphorylase
deficiency *see* Glycogen storage
disease V
Muscular dystrophy   165–166
Myasthenia congenita *see*
Myasthenia gravis
Myasthenia gravis   167–168
Myasthenic syndrome   169
Myelofibrosis *see* Bone marrow
failure

Myopathy — Carnitine deficiency 170
Myopathy — nemaline *see* Nemaline myopathy
Myotonia atrophica *see* Myotonica dystrophia
Myotonia congenita 171
Myotonica dystrophia (adult type) 172–173
Myotonica dystrophia (congenital) 174
Myotonic dystrophy *see* Myotonica dystrophia
Myxoedema *see* Hypothyroidism

Nemaline myopathy 175
Neonatal myasthenia gravis *see* Myasthenia gravis
Neurofibromatosis 176–177

Obesity 178–180
Occipital encephalocoele 181
Ocular muscular dystrophy 182
Ocular myopathy *see* Ocular muscular dystrophy
Oculo-auriculovertebral dysplasia 183–184
Oculomandibulodyscephaly with hypotrichosis *see* Hallerman-Streiff syndrome
Ondine's curse *see* Apnoea — obstructive sleep
Ophthalmoplegia plus 185
Opitz Frias syndrome 186
Osteitis deformans 187
Osteogenesis imperfecta 188–189
Osteopathia hyperostotica sclerotisans multiplex infantalis *see* Engelmann's disease
Osteopetrosis 190

Pacemakers 191
Paget's disease of bone *see* Osteitis deformans
Painful bruising syndrome *see* Auto erythrocyte sensitisation syndrome
Pancytopaenia *see* Bone marrow failure
Paraganglionoma *see* Glomus jugulare
Paralysis — familial periodic *see* Familial periodic paralysis

Paralysis agitans *see* Parkinson's disease
Paramyotonia congenita 192
Paraplegia 193
Parkinson's disease 194
Paroxysmal nocturnal haemoglobinuria 195
Pemphigus and pemphigoid 196–197
Periarteritis nodosa *see* Polyarteritis nodosa
Peroneal muscular atrophy 198
Phaeochromocytoma 199–200
Pharyngeal teratoma 201
Phenylketonuria 202
Pickwickian syndrome *see* Apnoea — obstructive sleep
Pierre Robin syndrome *see* Mandibulofacial dysostosis
Pneumatosis cystoides intestinalis 203
Poliomyelitis *see* Amyotrophic lateral sclerosis
Polyarteritis nodosa 204
Polymyositis *see* Dermatomyositis
Pompe's disease *see* Glycogen storage disease II
Porphyria 205–206
Prader Labhart Willi syndrome *see* Prader Willi syndrome
Prader Willi syndrome 207–208
Pre-excitation syndrome *see* Wolff–Parkinson–White syndrome
Primary alveolar hypoventilation *see* Apnoea — Obstructive sleep
Primary lateral sclerosis *see* Amyotrophic lateral sclerosis
Prinzmetal's variant angina 209
Progeria 210
Progressive external ophthalmoplegia *see* Ophthalmoplegia plus
Progressive muscular atrophy *see* Amyotrophic lateral sclerosis
Progressive muscular dystrophy *see* Muscular dystrophy
Progressive ophthalmoplegia *see* Ophthalmoplegia plus
Progressive systemic sclerosis *see* Scleroderma
Prolonged QT syndrome 211–212
Protein C deficiency 213
Prune Belly syndrome 214–215
Pseudobulbar palsy *see* Amyotrophic

lateral sclerosis
Pseudohaemophilia *see* Von
  Willebrand's disease
Pseudohypertrophic muscular
  dystrophy *see* Muscular dystrophy
Pseudohyperparathyroidism *see*
  Hypercalcaemia
Pseudomyasthenia *see* Myasthenic
  syndrome
Pseudoxanthoma elasticum 216
Pulmonary fibrosis (secondary to
  antineoplastics) 217
Pulseless disease *see* Takayasu's
  arteritis
Pyruvate dehydrogenase deficiency
  218

QT syndrome *see* Prolonged QT
  syndrome

Receptoma *see* Glomus jugulare
Refsum's disease *see* Heredopathia
  atactica polyneuritiformis
Renal tubular acidosis *see* Fanconi
  syndrome
Reye's syndrome 219
Rheumatoid arthritis 220
Riley-Day syndrome *see*
  Dysautonomia
Romano-Ward syndrome *see*
  Prolonged QT syndrome
Rotor syndrome *see* Bilirubin
  metabolism — abnormalities
Rubenstein-Taybi syndrome 221

Sanfilippo syndrome *see*
  Mucopolysaccharidosis III
Sarcoidosis 222–223
Scheie's disease *see*
  Mucopolysaccharidosis I S
Scleroderma 224–225
Sheehan's syndrome 226
Short stature *see* Dwarfism
Shy-Drager syndrome 227–228
Siamese twins *see* Conjoined twins
Sickle cell disease and trait 230–231
Sick sinus syndrome 229
Silver syndrome *see* Dwarfism
Sipple's syndrome *see* Apudomas
Sjogren's syndrome 232
Skeletal dysplasia *see* Dwarfism
Sleep apnoea syndrome *see*
  Apnoea — obstructive sleep

Sleep paralysis 233
Spinal cord transection *see* Paraplegia
Spinal muscular atrophy 234–235
Spondyloepiphyseal dysplasia *see*
  Dwarfism
Spondylometepiphyseal dysplasia
  236
Spongiform encephalopathy —
  subacute *see* Creutzfeldt-Jakob
  disease
Sprengel's deformity 237
Startle disease *see* Stiff baby
  syndrome
Steinart's disease *see* Myotonica
  dystrophia
Stevens Johnson syndrome *see*
  Erythema multiforme
Stiff baby syndrome 238
Still's disease *see* Juvenile chronic
  polyarthritis
Stokes Adams attacks *see* Heart block
Sturge-Weber syndrome 239
Subacute necrotising
  encephalomyelopathy *see* Leigh's
  syndrome
Subclavian steal syndrome 240
Systemic lupus erythematosis 241
Systemic sclerosis *see* Scleroderma

Takayasu's arteritis 242
Testicular feminisation syndrome
  244
Thallassaemia 245
Thomsen's disease *see* Myotonia
  congenita
Thrombocytopaenia *see* Bone
  marrow failure
Thrombocytopaenic purpura 246
Thrombotic thrombocytopaenic
  purpura *see* Thrombocytopaenic
  purpura
Thymic hypoplasia syndrome *see*
  DiGeorge syndrome
Thyrotoxicosis *see* Hyperthyroidism
Torsion dystonia 247–248
Tourette syndrome 249
Tracheal cylindroma *see* Tracheal
  reconstruction
Tracheal reconstruction 250–251
Tracheobronchial malacia *see*
  Tracheomegaly
Tracheobronchiomegaly *see*
  Tracheomegaly
Tracheobronchopathica

osteochondroplastica 252
Tracheomegaly 253
Transplanted heart 254–255
Treacher-Collins syndrome *see*
  Mandibulofacial dysostosis
Trismus — pseudocamptodactyly
  syndrome *see* Dutch-Kentucky
  syndrome
Trisomy 21 256
Trypanosomiasis *see* American
  trypanosomiasis
Turner's syndrome 257

Urticaria pigmentosa *see*
  Mastocytosis
Uveoparotid fever *see* Heerfordts
  syndrome

Variant angina, Prinzmetal *see*
  Prinzmetal's variant angina
Vipomas *see* Apudomas 22
Von Gierke's disease *see* Glycogen
  storage disease I
Von Hippel-Lindau syndrome 258

Von Recklinghausen's disease *see*
  Neurofibromatosis
Von Willebrand's disease 259

WDHA syndrome *see* Apudomas
Weaver's syndrome 260
Welander muscular atrophy *see*
  Distal muscular dystrophy
Werdnig-Hoffmann disease *see*
  Spinal muscular atrophy
Wermer's syndrome *see* Apudomas
Werner-Morrison syndrome *see*
  Apudomas
Whistling face syndrome *see*
  Freeman-Sheldon syndrome
Windmill-Vane-Hand syndrome *see*
  Freeman-Sheldon syndrome
Wiskott-Aldrich syndrome 261
Wolff-Parkinson-White syndrome
  262

Zollinger-Ellison syndrome *see*
  Apudomas